Valerie DeLaune's Trigger Point Therapy for Headaches and Migraines *delivers highly effective, safe, and easy-to-learn self-care techniques that will help the reader ease pain and improve body function. I can therefore confidently recommend this book to anyone who suffers from stubborn head, neck, shoulder, or back pain and dysfunction."*

—Bernard L. Gladieux, Jr., president of The Pressure Positive Company

Headaches are among the most common ailments, and any resource to help sufferers is a welcome addition. With this book, Ms. Delaune gives you a tool you can use to help yourself. The photos are excellent, and the text is very easy for anyone to understand.

—Honora Lee Wolfe, certified acupuncturist and author of *Managing Menopause Naturally with Chinese Medicine* and *Points for Profit*

Trigger Point Therapy for Headaches & Migraines

YOUR SELF-TREATMENT WORKBOOK FOR PAIN RELIEF

Valerie DeLaune, L.Ac.

New Harbinger Publications, Inc.

Publisher's Note

This publication is designed to provide accurate and authoritative information in regard to the subject matter covered. It is sold with the understanding that the publisher is not engaged in rendering psychological, financial, legal, or other professional services. If expert assistance or counseling is needed, the services of a competent professional should be sought.

Distributed in Canada by Raincoast Books

Copyright © 2008 by Valerie DeLaune, LAC
                New Harbinger Publications, Inc.
                5674 Shattuck Avenue
                Oakland, CA 94609
                www.newharbinger.com

Cover design by Amy Shoup
Text design by Michele Waters-Kermes
Acquired by Jess O'Brien
Edited by Jasmine Star

Library of Congress Cataloging in Publication Data on file

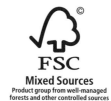

FSC

Mixed Sources

Product group from well-managed
forests and other controlled sources

Cert no. SW-COC-002283
www.fsc.org
© 1996 Forest Stewardship Council

10   09   08

10   9   8   7   6   5   4   3   2

Contents

Foreword

At the same time that health care spending is spiraling out of control, millions of Americans are in chronic pain, with head pain being one of the most common pain syndromes. According to statistics, the quality of health care in the United States is among the worst of any industrial country, and yet we pay the most for that care in both absolute and per capita terms. In addition, many of our conventional interventions cause more problems than they help. In fact, we are in the unenviable position of paying more money for less health and longevity than any other country in the world. In terms of resolving this health care crisis, the government, insurance companies, drug companies, medical centers, and most patients seem to be stuck going nowhere.

But against this backdrop, the tide has been turning in the form of quiet health care revolution few people have noticed. Patients are now more likely to see natural practitioners than anyone would have guessed before surveys by David Eisenberg, director of Harvard Medical School's Division for Research and Education in Complementary and Integrative Medical Therapies. In 1982, John Naisbitt, a best-selling author in the field of future studies, predicted there would be a megatrend of low-tech, high-touch approaches in health care, something David Eisenberg's surveys support, but in reality, the watershed event preceded even him by decades.

Between World Wars I and II, Dr. Janet Travell, a young female cardiologist, was working at a major American medical center. She was assigned patients who had recovered from heart attacks but were still experiencing chest and left shoulder or arm pain even though EKGs and other tests indicated no heart problems. These patients were considered cranks or, in the vernacular of the day, hypochondriacs. Perhaps Dr. Travell was assigned these patients because, being female, it was thought she wasn't capable of "serious" work. However, she not only worked them up using standard cardiological procedures, she also examined and palpated the painful areas and systematically mapped her results. After determining that most of the pain was originating from the patients' pectoralis minor muscle, she used a hypodermic needle to break up those points that triggered the pain. Later on, she studied other anatomical areas and developed techniques to treat these areas of muscle that referred pain to other regions of the body.

Dr. Travell devoted her life to this field of study and published authoritative texts on the subject. Her books have informed a new era of health care—one in which nonphysicians have emerged as health care providers, giving patients a wider range of choices in care. Tenets of alternative health care include treating the entire person, not just the symptoms, and involving patients in their own care. In terms of trigger points, practitioners have developed many methods of self-treatment that patients can easily learn and use. Finally, patients are becoming full participants in the delivery of their own care.

Most people have functional pain patterns, meaning pain that can't be traced to a cause such as fractures, infections, cancer, or significant changes that show on imaging studies. Functional pain results from misusing the body mechanically, locking emotions into the body by tightening areas, or improper nutrition. What is now called CAM (complementary and alternative medicine) but is better recognized as natural medicine is the most effective approach to solving these functional problems. Approaches such as the self-help techniques offered by Valerie DeLaune in this book could dramatically reduce the need for pharmaceutical and surgical interventions. Beyond lowering health care costs, this approach ultimately helps make people healthier by treating the whole person and addressing the root causes of symptoms. It also has virtually no side effects.

In this book, and in her earlier work, Valerie DeLaune has made the concepts and methods of Dr. Travell more accessible to the layperson. Her approach allows people with chronic pain, but without extensive anatomical and physiological knowledge, to successfully help themselves. Read, study, and follow the advice in this book and it will likely change your life for the better in a big way.

—Steven Lavitan, DC, L.Ac.

Acknowledgments

Approximately 38 percent of the human population is in pain at any given time. Although 30 percent of patients seen in a general physician's practice are there due to pain caused by trigger points (Simons 2003), there is still very little emphasis in medical school on muscle pain and trigger points. Thankfully, a few pioneers have worked endlessly to research trigger points, document referral patterns and other symptoms, and bring all of that information to medical practitioners and the general public.

This book would not have been possible without the lifework of Dr. Janet Travell and Dr. David Simons, and my neuromuscular therapy instructor, Jeanne Aland, who introduced me to the books written by Doctors Travell and Simons. Both Dr. Travell and Jeanne Aland have passed on, but I know that I and all of my patients are eternally grateful for their hard work and dedication. Their work lives on through the hundreds of thousands of patients who have gotten relief because of their research and willingness to train others.

Dr. Janet Travell

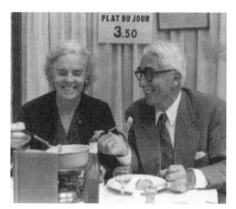

Janet Travell Powell and Jack Powell, 1956. Photo courtesy of Virginia Street.

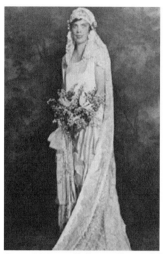

Janet Travell Powell, 1929. Photo courtesy of Virginia Street.

Dr. Travell was born in 1901 and followed in her father's footsteps to become a doctor. She initially specialized in cardiology but soon became interested in pain relief, as had her father. She joined her father's practice, taught at Cornell University Medical College, and pioneered and researched new pain treatments, including trigger point injections. In her private practice, she began treating Senator John F. Kennedy, who at the time was using crutches due to crippling back pain and was almost unable to walk down just a few stairs. This was at a time when television was just beginning to bring images of politicians into the nation's living rooms, and it had become important for presidential candidates to appear physically fit. Being on crutches probably would have cost President Kennedy the election.

Dr. Travell became the first female White House physician, and after President Kennedy died she stayed on to treat President Johnson. She resigned a year and a half later to return to her passions: teaching, lecturing, and writing about chronic myofascial pain. She continued to work into her nineties and died at the age of ninety-five on August 1, 1997.

Dr. David G. Simons

Dr. Simons, who started out his career as an aerospace physician, met Dr. Travell when she lectured at the School of Aerospace Medicine at Brooks Air Force Base in Texas in the 1960s. He soon teamed up with Dr. Travell and began researching the international literature for any references to the treatment of pain. He discovered there were a few others out there who were also discovering trigger points but using different terminology. He studied and documented the physiology of trigger points in both laboratory and clinical settings and tried to find scientific explanations for trigger

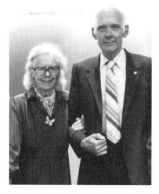

Dr. Janet Travell and Dr. David G. Simons, 1977. Photo courtesy of Dr. David G. Simons.

points. Together, Doctors Travell and Simons produced a comprehensive two-volume text on the causes and treatment of trigger points, written for physicians.

Other Thanks

Many additional researchers have contributed to the study of trigger points, and many doctors and other practitioners have taken the time to learn about trigger points and give that information to their patients. I would like to acknowledge all of them for their role in alleviating pain by making this important information available.

My editors Jess Beebe, Jess O'Brien, and Jasmine Star did an excellent job providing organizational suggestions and inspiring me to make each revision even better. I would also like to thank Art Sutch, Skip Gray, and Don Douglas for the still photography, David Ham for being the model in the referral pattern photos, and Laura Lucas and Sarah Olsen for graphic design work. Virginia Street (Janet Travell's daughter) and Dr. Simons provided some of the photos.

I owe many thanks to the thousands of patients and some practitioners who shared with me what worked for them so that I could share that information with you. But most of all, I would like to thank Sasha the dog for waiting patiently while I worked too many hours to finish this book.

Introduction

If you've picked up this book, chances are that you suffer from headaches that occur frequently or that are intense or debilitating. You're certainly not alone; by some estimates, forty-five million Americans suffer from chronic, recurring headaches, and headaches are responsible for more missed days of work and school than any other cause (Cleveland Clinic 2007). Despite this, there's seldom a magic bullet for curing headaches. In part, this is because the causes of headaches are often wide-ranging and complex. Until the underlying or perpetuating causes are addressed, they usually recur. Headaches can be an intractable problem because some of the causes are seldom recognized.

This book will help you sort through the potential causes of your headaches and offer self-help tips to address those perpetuating factors. In part I, you will learn about what *trigger points* are, general information about treating them, and their role in causing headaches, migraines, and temporomandibular joint dysfunction. Part II will help you identify perpetuating factors that are causing your pain and causing trigger points to form, such as poor body mechanics, poorly designed furniture, dietary factors, stress, sleep problems, and acute and chronic illnesses. It will also give you suggestions for how to eliminate those causes. Part III will teach you where to find trigger points and how to treat them by applying pressure and stretching the muscles.

My Background

I attended massage school in 1989 and learned Swedish massage. I learned to give a very good general massage, but trying to solve a patient's muscular problems was often frustrating and elusive. I saw a class on neuromuscular therapy (which combines a type of deep tissue massage with treating trigger points) in the Heartwood Institute catalog and was very intrigued by the description. I attended the class in 1991, taught by Jeanne Aland, and it completely changed my approach to treating patients.

The most important thing I learned about trigger points during that class is that they refer pain to other areas in fairly consistent patterns. For example, pain felt on your forehead may be coming from a muscle in your forehead, but it may also be coming from a trigger point located in muscles on the front of your neck. Knowledge of referral patterns gives us a starting point of where to look for the trigger points that are actually causing the pain. Once I learned this, I was able to start solving problems consistently, even in cases where people had been led to believe they would have to live with their pain.

I bought Janet Travell and David Simons's first volume on the upper half of the body, *Myofascial Pain and Dysfunction: The Trigger Point Manual* (Travell and Simons 1983), and then anxiously awaited completion of the second volume on the lower half of the body, which came out in 1992. While the neuromuscular therapy class taught me about trigger point referral patterns and how to search for and treat trigger points, the books taught me so much more—about causative (perpetuating) factors, symptoms other than pain referral patterns, and some self-treatment techniques I could teach to patients.

Over my years of treating thousands of patients, I have added my own observations and developed a variety of self-help techniques. In 1999 I received my master's degree in acupuncture, and since then I've been specializing in treating pain syndromes and trigger points with acupuncture.

How This Book Is Organized

Of the pain syndromes I treat, the most common are headaches, upper back pain, and neck pain. As you read through the book, you'll learn how these are related to each other, and how muscular problems can play a very significant role in headaches, even migraine-type headaches. Because trigger points are so often involved in headaches, learning self-treatment techniques is critical to obtaining long-term relief in the majority of cases of headache pain.

Part I offers background information on trigger points and why it's important to treat pain as soon as possible. Part I also describes the various types of headaches and discusses their causes and how trigger points can be involved in each type. Temporomandibular joint (TMJ) problems often play a role in headaches, too, but many people don't suspect a link or even realize that they have a TMJ problem.

Part II of this book will help you identify the factors that are pertinent to your particular set of circumstances and symptoms. Many things cause and keep trigger points activated: poor posture, poorly designed furniture, chronic and acute illness, emotional factors, and poor diet, to name a few. These will have to be addressed in conjunction with self-help techniques. Headaches often have causative factors in addition to trigger points. For example, failing to drink enough water will not directly cause and perpetuate trigger points, but it can cause or contribute to causing your headaches.

Part III provides instructions for locating the muscles that potentially contain trigger points, applying pressure to those trigger points, and stretching the muscles. Chapter 8 describes treatment guidelines in detail, and chapter 9 provides a guide indicating which muscle chapters you will want to peruse as potential contributors to your headaches or temporomandibular pain. Chapters 10 through 18 help you identify the specific muscles that are causing your headache and TMJ pain. They contain lists of common symptoms for specific trigger points, offer helpful hints, and describe self-treatment techniques and stretches.

How to Use This Book

Once you've read part I, start reading part II, on trigger point causes and perpetuating factors. However, identifying the perpetuating factors that apply to you—and then eliminating them—may take some time. You'll want to apply pressure to your trigger points in the meantime, so go ahead and start on part III of the book before you've finished part II. But before you start using the self-treatments described in chapters 10 through 18, carefully read through the treatment guidelines in chapter 8 and then consult chapter 9 for guidance on how to identify which muscles are causing your headaches. Be sure to come back and read through all of part II as soon as you can. In all likelihood, a combination of these perpetuating factors is involved. You won't get lasting relief from your trigger points (and thus from your headaches) until you address the things that are causing and aggravating your trigger points, so it's important to read through all of part II and carefully consider whether each factor could possibly apply to you.

This is not a quick fix! There is no such thing as resolving your pain in fifteen minutes or less in five easy steps with any technique. I recommend that, if possible, you have your trigger points identified by a practitioner who has been trained in treating trigger points, such as a neuromuscular massage therapist or possibly a physical therapist, and use the book to supplement their work. In my experience, people who do self-treatments at home in addition to receiving professional treatments weekly improve at least five times faster than those who receive only professional treatments.

Unfortunately, you may not have the option of locating a professional to help you. It could take longer for you to locate trigger points without the guidance of a professional, but with this book you will most likely be able to locate the trigger points yourself. You will need to read the chapters, search for trigger points in your muscles, and use the self-treatment techniques on a regular basis until your pain is resolved. Ask yourself, "Is it worth some of my time to resolve my pain?" If the answer is yes, then you will find the information in this book very helpful.

Be sure to set realistic goals. Focus on a few muscles at a time unless there is a reason that you need to work on several together. Setting unrealistic goals can lead to discouragement and cause you to give up. It's better to pick just a few things and do them well rather than rush through a greater number of self-help techniques or suggestions and do them poorly. You probably won't be able to apply pressure on five different muscles and stretch them, learn proper breathing and posture, replace all your furniture at work, change your diet, and start walking every day all in the first week. Pace yourself so that this is an enjoyable process, and work on the perpetuating factors over time.

If you're working with a practitioner, they should be able to help you prioritize what needs to be done in order of most importance. If your practitioner is giving you too many things to do at once, be sure to tell them that you are overwhelmed and need to set priorities. Giving a patient too many assignments is all too easy for a practitioner to do when they are first out of school and brimming with many useful ideas and suggestions.

There are hundreds of suggestions in this book. As you read through part II, on perpetuating factors, and the "Helpful Hints" in the muscle chapters you have identified as potentially causing your pain referral patterns, highlight anything that might be pertinent to your situation. Then plan to devote some time to accomplishing your goals. Resolving pain is like detective work—what causes *your* pain and also what resolves it will be a combination of factors unique to you. This book gives you numerous tools for your process of self-discovery on the road to relief from pain.

Part I

TRIGGER POINTS, HEADACHES, AND TEMPOROMANDIBULAR JOINT DYSFUNCTION

If you're suffering from headaches, all too often you may be diagnosed with general terms such as tension headache, migraine, or TMJ pain without the true cause being identified. Often the cause is trigger points in one or more muscles, but the diagnosing practitioner is unfamiliar with trigger points. Trigger points can play a very large role in most types of chronic and acute headaches, as well as temporomandibular joint problems, which means you may be able to get a great deal of relief, or even complete relief, by working on trigger points and eliminating perpetuating factors.

Your headache, migraine, and TMJ pain is likely treatable. The sooner you start doing the self-help techniques and possibly receiving treatment from a practitioner, the sooner you will get relief. This is important, since untreated pain can create an escalating cycle that makes the pain more chronic and more resistant to treatment.

Chapter 1

What Are Trigger Points?

In this chapter you'll learn what trigger points are, how they form, and what it feels like when they're pressed. You'll also learn how they refer pain to areas of the body remote from the trigger point itself, what symptoms they can cause other than pain, and what happens when they're left untreated.

Characteristics of Trigger Points

Muscle is the largest organ in the human body, typically accounting for almost 50 percent of the body's weight. There are approximately four hundred muscles in the human body (surprisingly, there are individual variations), and any one of them can develop trigger points, potentially causing referred pain and dysfunction. Symptoms can range from intolerable, agonizing pain to painless restriction of movement and distortion of posture.

Knots, Tight Bands, and Tenderness in the Muscle

Muscles consist of many muscle cells, or fibers, bundled together and surrounded by connective tissue. Each fiber contains numerous myofibrils. Most skeletal muscles contain approximately one thousand to two thousand myofibrils, and each myofibril consists of a chain of sarcomeres connected end-to-end. Muscular contractions take place in the sarcomere. When a trigger point is present, numerous sarcomeres are contracted into a small thickened area and the rest of the sarcomeres in the myofibril are stretched thin. Several of these contractures in the same area are probably what we feel as a "knot" or "tight band" in the muscle. These muscle fibers are not available for use because they are already contracted, which is why you cannot condition (strengthen) a muscle that contains trigger points.

When pressed, trigger points are usually very tender. The sustained contraction of the fibril probably leads to the release of sensitizing *neurochemicals* (body substances that affect the nervous system), producing the pain that is felt when the trigger point is pressed. Pain intensity levels can vary depending on the amount of stress placed on the muscles. The intensity of pain can also vary in response to flare-ups of any of the other perpetuating factors, such as emotional factors, illnesses, and insomnia.

Healthy muscles usually do not contain knots or tight bands, are not tender to pressure, and, when not in use, feel soft and pliable to the touch, not like the hard and dense muscles found in people with chronic pain. People often tell me their muscles feel hard and dense because they work out and do strengthening exercises, but healthy muscles feel soft and pliable when not being used, even if you work out.

Referred Pain

Trigger points may refer pain both in the local area and/or to other areas of the body, and the most common patterns have been well documented and diagrammed. These are called *referral patterns*. Approximately half of the time, trigger points are not located in the same place where you feel symptoms. This means that if you only work on the areas where you feel pain, you probably won't get relief. In part III, you'll find illustrations of common pain referral patterns that you can compare with your pain patterns, and this will help you figure out where the trigger point or points causing your pain are located. Unless you know that you need to search in that location, you probably won't get relief. For example, trigger points in the upper portion of the trapezius muscle (between the neck and the shoulder) can cause headache pain in the temples, the base of the skull, in the angle of the jaw, and possibly above the ear and over the eye.

When you apply pressure to the trigger point, you can often reproduce the referred pain or other symptoms, but being unable to reproduce the referred pain or other symptoms by applying pressure does not rule out involvement of that specific trigger point. Try treating the trigger points that could be causing the problem anyway, and if you improve, even temporarily, assume that one of the trigger points you worked on is indeed at least part of the problem. For this reason, don't work on all the possible trigger points in one session, since you won't know which trigger point treated actually gave you relief.

Referred tingling, numbness, or burning sensations are more likely due to trigger points constricting around or putting pressure on a nerve. For example, the sciatic nerve runs either under or through the piriformis muscle in the gluteal area, and trigger points in the piriformis muscle can compress the sciatic nerve, causing a pseudosciatic pain that mimics true sciatica (Travell and Simons 1983).

Weakness and Muscle Fatigue

Trigger points cause weakness and loss of coordination of the involved muscles, along with an inability of the muscles to tolerate use. Many people take this as a sign that they need to strengthen the weak muscles, but if the trigger points aren't inactivated first, strengthening (conditioning) exercises will likely encourage the surrounding muscles to do the work instead of the muscle containing the trigger point, further weakening and deconditioning the muscle containing trigger points.

Muscles containing trigger points are fatigued more easily and don't return to a relaxed state as quickly when use of the muscle ceases. In addition, trigger points may cause other muscles to tighten and become weak and fatigued in the areas where you experience the referred pain, and also cause a generalized tightening of an area as a response to pain.

Other Symptoms

Trigger points can cause symptoms not normally associated with muscular problems, such as swelling, ringing in the ears, loss of balance, dizziness, urinary frequency, buckling knees, abnormal sweating, and tearing of the eyes. You may suffer from stiff joints, fatigue, generalized weakness, twitching, trembling, and areas of numbness or other odd sensations. For example, the sternocleidomastoid muscle, in addition to causing a tension-type headache, can also cause dizziness, nausea, sinus congestion, eyelid twitching, hearing problems, eye problems, a chronic sore throat, and other symptoms. It probably wouldn't occur to you that these symptoms could be caused by a trigger point in a muscle.

Active Phase Versus Latent Phase

A trigger point can be in either an active or a latent phase, depending on how irritated it is. If the trigger point is *active*, it will refer pain or other sensations and limit range of motion. If the trigger point is *latent*, it may cause only a decreased range of motion and weakness, but not pain. The more frequent and intense your headaches, the greater the number of active trigger points you're likely to have.

Trigger points that start with some impact to the muscle, such as an injury, are usually active initially. Poor posture or poor body mechanics, repetitive use, or a nerve root irritation can also form active trigger points. Active trigger points may at some point stop referring pain and become latent. However, these latent trigger points can easily become active again, which may lead you to believe you're experiencing a new problem when in fact an old problem—perhaps even something you've forgotten about—is being reaggravated. Latent trigger points can be reactivated by overuse, overstretching, or muscle chilling. Any of the perpetuating factors discussed in part II can activate previously latent trigger points and make you more prone to developing new trigger points initiated by impacts to muscles.

Latent trigger points can also develop gradually without being active first, and you don't even know they are there. In a study of thirteen healthy people with the same eight muscles examined in each (Simons 2003), two people had latent trigger points in seven of those muscles, one person had latent trigger points in six muscles, three had latent trigger points in five muscles, two had latent trigger points in three muscles, two had latent trigger points in two muscles, two had latent trigger points in one muscle, and only one person didn't have latent trigger points in any of the eight muscles! This means that most people have at least some latent trigger points, which can easily be converted to active trigger points. This also means that some people are more prone to develop problems with muscular pain than others (Simons 2003).

Locations of Trigger Points Within the Muscles

Trigger points tend to form where the nerve ending that causes the muscle to contract attaches to the muscle fiber, generally in the middle of the muscle fiber. These are called *central myofascial trigger points*. Trigger points also tend to form at the muscle's attachments; these are called *attachment trigger points*. Since you may not know where the middle of the muscle fiber is or where the attachments are, I recommend that you look at the muscle drawings in part III and try to work on the *entire* muscle so that you won't miss treating any trigger points within the muscle.

A *primary*, or *key*, trigger point can cause a *satellite*, or *secondary*, trigger point to develop in a different muscle. It may form because it lies within the referral zone of the primary trigger point. Alternatively, the muscle with the satellite trigger point may be overloaded because it's substituting for the muscle with the primary trigger point, or it may be countering the tension in the muscle with the primary trigger point. When doing self-treatments, be aware that some of your trigger points may be satellite trigger points, in which case you won't be able to treat them effectively until the primary trigger points causing them have been treated. Part III offers guidance in this regard.

What Happens When You Leave Trigger Points Untreated?

When people first develop some kind of pain problem, they usually wait to see if it will go away. Sometimes it does, and sometimes it doesn't. The problem with "waiting to see" is that when trigger points are left untreated, muscles can be damaged, and eventually changes to the central nervous system can lead to a vicious cycle of pain. This central nervous system involvement probably explains why you are experiencing chronic headaches and pain.

Damage to the Muscle Fibers

Remember how trigger points cause portions of the myofibril to stay contracted? If this goes on too long, the myofibril may break in the middle, causing it to retract to each end and leave an empty shell in the middle. Muscle fibers damaged in this way cannot be repaired and will never be available for use again (Simons, Travell, and Simons 1999).

Facilitated Nerve Pathways

When pain travels repeatedly through the same nerve, it will cause a *facilitated nerve pathway*. This means that any time a new injury or other stress occurs in an area where pain was previously experienced, pain will tend to travel along the same nerve pathway again. Remember that the most common patterns have been well documented and diagrammed? A facilitated nerve pathway can cause the pain referral to deviate from the most commonly found pattern. It may also cause trigger points in several muscles in the region to refer pain to the same area, making it all the harder to determine the actual source of the referred pain. This means you can't absolutely rule out the role of a potential trigger point based only on consideration of common referral patterns, since other factors may cause you to have an *uncommon* referral pattern. The more intense the earlier pain and the more intense the emotions associated with it, the more likely the facilitated nerve pathway will cause deviation from the most common referral patterns (Simons, Travell, and Simons 1999).

Central Nervous System Sensitization

Recent research (Borg-Stein and Simons 2002) has shown that certain types of nerve receptors in muscles relay information to neurons located within part of the gray matter of the spinal cord. The pain is amplified there and then is relayed to areas of other muscles, thereby expanding the region of pain beyond the initially affected area.

Once this part of the central nervous system is involved, or sensitized, in this way (called *central sensitization*), the persistent pain leads to long-term or permanent changes in these neurons, which affect adjacent neurons through *neurotransmitters* (chemical substances that are produced and secreted by a neuron and then diffuse across *synapses*, or small gaps, between neurons, causing excitation or inhibition of another neuron). This may also cause the part of the nervous system that would normally counteract pain to malfunction and fail to do its job. The longer pain goes untreated, the greater the number of neurons that get involved, and the more muscles they affect, causing pain in new areas, and in turn causing more neurons to get involved . . . and the bigger the problem keeps getting, leading to the likelihood that the pain is going to turn into a chronic problem. The sooner pain is treated, the less likely it will become a permanent problem with widespread muscle involvement and central nervous system changes.

Sensitization of the Opposite Side of the Body

You may be surprised to discover that the same area on the opposite side of your body is also tender to pressure, even though that side isn't otherwise painful. Over half of the time, the opposite side is actually more tender with pressure. Unless it is a recent injury, it's typical for both sides to eventually get involved (for example, if the right midback is painful, there are likely to be tender points on the left midback). For that reason, I almost always work on both sides, and I recommend that you do self-treatments on both sides.

This observation has been supported by a study in which the researchers used needle electrodes placed in the same spot on both sides of the neck or back to record muscle electrical activity (Audette, Wang, and Smith 2004). When an active trigger point was stimulated on one side of the body, it induced electrical muscle activity on the corresponding opposite side. Latent trigger points did not produce the same results. This further supports the concept of central nervous system sensitization, which would cause corresponding trigger points to form on the opposite side of the body over time.

How Trigger Points Form

Trigger points may form after a sudden trauma or injury, or they may develop gradually. Common initiating and perpetuating factors are mechanical stresses, injuries, nutritional problems, emotional factors, sleep problems, acute or chronic infections, organ dysfunction and disease, and other medical conditions. Part II goes into detail about these causes and perpetuators of trigger points.

Part of the current hypothesis about the mechanism responsible for the formation of trigger points is the energy crisis component theory. The *sarcoplasmic reticulum*, a part of each cell, is responsible for storing and releasing ionized calcium. The type of nerve ending that causes the muscle fiber to contract is called a *motor end plate*. This nerve ending releases *acetylcholine*, a neurotransmitter that tells the sarcoplasmic reticulum to release calcium, and then the muscle fiber contracts. If it is operating normally, when contraction of the muscle fiber is no longer needed, the nerve ending stops releasing acetylcholine and the calcium pump in the sarcoplasmic reticulum returns calcium into the sarcoplasmic reticulum. If a trauma occurs or there is a large increase in the motor end plate's release of acetylcholine, an excessive amount of calcium can be released by the sarcoplasmic reticulum, causing a maximal contracture of a segment of muscle, leading to a maximal demand for energy and impairment of local circulation. If circulation is impeded, the calcium pump doesn't get the fuel and oxygen it needs to pump calcium back into the sarcoplasmic reticulum, so the muscle fiber continues to contract.

The areas at the ends of the muscle fibers (either at the bone or where the muscle attaches to a tendon) also become tender as the attachments are stressed by the contraction in the center of the fiber (Simons, Travell, and Simons 1999). Once the central nervous system has been sensitized, various substances are released: *histamine* (a compound that causes dilation and permeability of blood vessels), *serotonin* (a neurotransmitter that constricts blood vessels), *bradykinin* (a hormone that dilates peripheral blood vessels and increases small blood vessel permeability), and *substance P* (a compound involved in the regulation of the pain threshold). These substances stimulate the nervous system to release even more acetylcholine locally, adding to the perpetuation of the dysfunctional cycle (Borg-Stein and Simons 2002). This vicious cycle continues until some sort of outside intervention stretches the contracted portion of the muscle fiber. Anxiety and nervous tension also increase *autonomic nervous system* activity (the part of the nervous system that controls the release of acetylcholine, along with involuntary functions of blood vessels and glands), which commonly aggravates trigger points and their associated symptoms (Simons 2004).

Conclusion

Trigger points are tender when pressed, and the multiple contractures forming the trigger point may feel like a small lump in the muscle. Healthy muscles don't contain trigger points, and they don't feel tender with pressure. If trigger points are left untreated, the damage to the muscle cells can be irreparable and can even cause long-term changes in the central nervous system, leading to a self-perpetuating cycle of trigger points, pain, and muscular damage. Trigger points can cause symptoms other than pain, which should be taken into consideration and may help you determine which muscles contain trigger points. This is particularly important when the referral pattern deviates from the common pattern, making the location of the trigger points harder to determine.

In the next chapter you'll learn more about treating trigger points and when you should see a doctor.

Chapter 2

Treating Trigger Points

It is important to treat trigger points as soon as possible so that they are less likely to cause chronic pain problems. Part III outlines general guidelines for self-treatment and teaches you how to treat the trigger points involved in headaches. The purpose of this chapter is to explain the importance of prompt treatment, and also to give you some idea of what to expect from treatment and when you might need to consult a doctor.

Headache and Migraine Pain Is Treatable

People often assume that if a parent had the same type of condition, it must be genetic and they'll just have to learn to live with it. It is true that if one parent has migraines you're more likely to get migraines, and if both parents get migraines this increases your chances even more; however, at this time there is no known biological link, just a statistical correlation. While it may or may not be true that people's headaches are genetic, I never operate on the assumption that they are, or that a condition can't be improved even if it is genetic. You learn many things from your parents—eating habits, exercise habits, how you deal with stressful situations, even posture and gestures—and all of these can influence your health.

I frequently hear that practitioners have told people things like "You're just getting older" or "You'll just have to learn to live with it." How depressing! I never assume I can't help someone, or that I can't think of someone to refer them to, such as a chiropractor, naturopath, or surgeon, who can help them. I've actually treated several fairly simple cases where the person had been told their only recourse was to learn to live with their pain only because the doctor didn't know about trigger points or was unwilling to refer to an "alternative" practitioner. Thankfully, that has been changing. New doctors are exposed to a wider range of alternatives in medical school, and some doctors who have been out of school for some time are getting excited about exploring other options.

In spite of being told that you have to learn to live with your medical condition, assume you can change it—at least until you have exhausted all treatment options.

The Importance of Prompt Treatment

So often, I hear patients say, "I kept thinking it would go away." Sometimes symptoms will go away in a few days and never return. But more often, the longer you wait to see if pain will go away, the more muscles become involved in the chain reaction of chronic pain and dysfunction. A muscle hurts and forms trigger points, then the area of referral (where you feel the pain or other symptoms) starts to hurt and tighten up and forms its own satellite trigger points, then *that* area refers pain somewhere else, and so on. Or the pain may improve for a while, but the trigger points are really just in an inactive phase and can readily become active and cause pain or other symptoms once again.

As explained in chapter 1, eventually there will be permanent structural damage to the muscle cells and sensitization of the central nervous system. The problem gets more complex the longer trigger points are left untreated, becoming more painful, more debilitating, more frustrating, and more time-consuming and expensive to treat. Plus, the longer you wait, the less likely you are to get complete relief—and the more likely it is that your trigger points will be reactivated chronically and periodically.

Breaking the Pain Cycle

Something starts to hurt, so you tense the area up. Then it hurts more, so the muscle tightens up more, perpetuating and escalating the cycle of pain. Any intervention that helps treat trigger points and eliminate perpetuating factors can help break the cycle: trigger point self-treatments, stretching, heat and/or ice, chiropractic or osteopathic treatments, massage, ultrasound, homeopathy, biofeedback, trigger point injections, counseling, and even analgesics.

People are often surprised that I support the use of analgesics, such as aspirin and ibuprofen, but anything that breaks the pain cycle as soon as possible helps prevent the symptoms from getting worse or affecting other muscles. Plus, analgesics can help you tolerate the initial stages of treatment if you are in extreme pain. But be aware that just because your pain level has decreased, this doesn't mean the trigger points are gone. You still need to seek treatment, preferably as soon as possible. Analgesics will most likely take the edge off the pain, but unless you plan to take them as a long-term solution, you also need to treat the source of the problem.

Muscle relaxants are of limited value for people with pain caused by trigger points because muscle spasms are not the cause of the pain. Also, these drugs first release tension in the muscles that provide *protective splinting* (the muscles that contract to compensate for or protect the weakened muscles containing the trigger points). Removing this protective splinting increases the load on the muscle containing trigger points and leads to additional pain.

Why Trigger Point Therapy Works

Massage and self-treatment of trigger points will allow muscle cells to start uptaking oxygen and nutrients and eliminating metabolic wastes again, the proper cell metabolism process. Also, by pressing on the trigger points and making it hurt a little bit more than it's already hurting, it causes your body to release pain-masking chemicals such as endorphins, thereby breaking the pain cycle.

How Long Will Therapy Take?

A question I commonly get when people begin therapy is "How long will it take?" My general rule of thumb is that the longer the condition has been going on and the more medical conditions (of any kind) that you have, the greater the number of muscles that will become involved, which means that treatment will be more complex and take longer. If you are perfectly healthy and have only a recent minor injury, you may not need long-term therapy.

A major factor in the amount of time it takes to get relief from symptoms is how diligently you perform self-treatments, and how accurately you identify your perpetuating factors (discussed in part II) and succeed in eliminating them. As I mentioned in the introduction, in my experience, people who do self-treatments at home in addition to receiving weekly professional treatments improve at least five times faster than those who only receive professional treatments. As Doctors Travell and Simons said, "Treatments that are done *to* the patient should be minimized and effort should be concentrated in teaching what can be done *by* the patient. . . . As patients exercise increasing control [over symptom management] they improve both physically and emotionally" (1992, 549).

I can usually give patients a pretty good indication of how many treatments they may need by the end of the second or third treatment, based on their medical condition, how their muscles feel to me, their diligence about self-treatment and working on perpetuating factors, and how much they have improved (or not) within the first few weeks. If you are seeing a practitioner, after a few weeks ask for an assessment of how long and how frequently the practitioner expects to see you.

A small percentage of people will get worse before they get better, mostly in complex cases. Or the pain may move around, or you may have the perception that the pain moved around only because the worst areas have improved and now you are noticing the next worse area more. I encourage you to stick with your treatments. If the self-treatments are uncomfortable, try to find ways to ease the discomfort, such as reducing the frequency of treatments or decreasing the amount of pressure. It's helpful to keep a journal or other record of your pain and other symptoms. Chapter 9 includes blank charts that you can photocopy and use to document your pain. This will help you determine whether you're making progress, even at times when you don't perceive any changes in your symptoms. Also seek feedback from people who are close to you. Often they will notice progress in your mobility and activity level, even if you aren't aware of it.

I've only had a few cases where I wasn't able to help patients, and in these cases the people were so frustrated (and understandably so) after seeing professional after professional and receiving little or no help that they only allowed me to treat them a few times before giving up, *even if they had improved*.

Sometimes patients get a little worse before they get better, especially in complex cases, making them inclined to give up easily in the initial stages of treatment. I encourage you to give any treatment you try some amount of time before you decide it isn't working, even if your condition initially gets worse. Most professionals have numerous tools in their bag, and if something isn't working, they can try something else. Just give them some time to learn your body and observe how you use it. However, if a practitioner doesn't seem to care or have time for you, then by all means look for someone who cares about you getting better.

When Should You See a Doctor?

If you can't get relief by using the self-help techniques in this book, you need to see a doctor. It may be that something other than trigger points is causing or contributing to your headaches or TMJ pain. X-rays and other diagnostic tests can identify some conditions that may cause headaches, including cracked teeth, anatomical abnormalities, and nerve root irritations. Referred symptoms due to trigger points can mimic other, more serious conditions or occur concurrently with them. It may take some investigation to determine the ultimate cause of the problem, which will determine how it can most effectively be treated.

You should see a doctor immediately to rule out serious conditions if you have pain in your head with any of the following symptoms:

- Your pain has a sudden onset or starts after a head injury.

- Your pain lasts for more than a few days.

- The intensity of pain is greater than your previous headaches, or the symptoms are different (changes can be an indication of a different, more serious cause).

- Your headaches start after age fifty.

- Your headaches are accompanied by a stiff neck, fever, seizures, convulsions, blurred vision or other vision changes, eye pain, ear pain, dizziness, mental confusion, disorientation, lack of alertness, speech difficulties, drowsiness, or muscle numbness, tingling, or weakness.

- Your headaches are triggered by coughing, bending, or lying down.

- Your headaches cause severe nausea or vomiting.

Hopefully your doctor will rule out any serious conditions. If you are diagnosed with headache, migraine, or temporomandibular joint (TMJ) pain, chances are you can relieve much or all of your pain with a combination of self-treatment of trigger points and treating and eliminating the perpetuating factors. Regardless of the diagnosis you receive from a medical doctor or dentist, my general treatment principle is the same: Identify and eliminate all the underlying causes to the extent possible, and treat the trigger points.

Conclusion

The most important thing to learn from this chapter is that you don't necessarily have to live with your pain. There are treatment options, even if your current practitioner isn't aware of all the options. Analgesics, such as ibuprofen, and use of heat and cold can help break the pain cycle, but they are not a substitute for treatment of trigger points and elimination of perpetuating factors. The length of treatment will depend on your individual medical condition and how long the condition has been going on, and your commitment to doing self-treatments and identifying and addressing perpetuating factors. You may possibly get worse before you get better. If you have any of the symptoms listed above or the self-help techniques in this book aren't helping, see a doctor.

The next chapter will address specific types of headaches, and the role of trigger points in causing and perpetuating headaches.

Chapter 3

Headaches and Migraines

Most people have had some headaches. Some people may have them frequently enough to be annoying, but their headaches are more of an inconvenience. For others, headaches can be mildly to severely debilitating. If this book is in your hands, chances are you are in the latter category. In the United States alone, more than forty-five million people have chronic headaches, or one in six people (Cleveland Clinic 2007). The rate of incidence varies from country to country.

Symptoms and Causes of Headaches

A headache is defined as aching or pain in one or more areas of the head or neck. Both the frequency and pain level can vary greatly. About 90 percent of all headaches fall into three categories: tension headaches, migraines, and cluster headaches. The remaining 10 percent fall into the category of secondary headaches (Healthcommunities.com 2002).

Tension Headaches

Tension headaches are by far the most common type of chronic headache. People who experience migraines typically also have tension headaches in between their migraines.

Symptoms of Tension Headaches

Tension headaches usually affect both sides of the head and last from thirty minutes to several days or more. They're usually characterized by a mild to moderate level of "pressing" pain or a dull, steady ache, though the intensity may also be severe. They may affect your ability to sleep soundly. They are not accompanied by the additional symptoms listed below that distinguish migraine headaches. Women are more likely than men to have tension headaches.

Causes of Tension Headaches

The most common causes of tension headaches are muscular problems and associated postural problems. Tension headaches are often aggravated by stress, anxiety, depression, fatigue, noise, and glare, but they can also be associated with arthritis, disk problems, or degenerative bone disease in the neck or spine.

Temporomandibular disorder (TMD) can also cause tension headaches. The temporomandibular joint (TMJ), located just in front of your ear, is the hinge joint that allows your jaw to open. A 1983 study found that people with TMD are twice as likely to get headaches compared to non-TMD control subjects (Kemper and Okeson 1983). Of the subjects in both groups who had headaches, the frequency and severity of headaches was higher in those with TMD. In fact, headaches are the most common symptom in people with TMJ problems. Usually this will be a tension-type headache, but sometimes it will be a combination of migraines and tension headaches.

A 1996 study reported that when subjects were asked to clench their teeth for a prolonged period, it induced a headache in 68 percent of the subjects who had chronic tension headaches, whereas a headache was triggered in only 16 percent of the nonheadache control group (Jensen and Olesen 1996). When muscles in and around the mouth are treated for trigger points, headache symptoms usually lessen.

TMJ problems will be addressed in greater detail in chapter 4.

Trigger Points and Central Sensitization in Tension Headaches

A study by Dr. Lars Bendtsen (2000) confirmed the role of central sensitization in chronic tension headaches. In a group of subjects who all suffered from chronic tension headaches, they asked each person to report pain levels as muscles in the neck and on the head were pressed. Certain muscles were tender even when the subject was not experiencing a headache at the time.

Bendtsen theorized that long-term inputs from trigger points eventually lead to central sensitization in specific areas of the spinal cord and brain stem, which in turn causes additional changes in the affected muscles, a self-perpetuating cycle that converts periodic headaches into chronic tension headaches. Because of this, even if the original initiating factor causing episodic headaches is eliminated, the trigger point-central sensitization cycle can continue and worsen on its own. Bendtsen also reported on another study, which indicated that subjects with chronic tension headaches feel pain in the body sooner than healthy control subjects and have a lower threshold for pain tolerance (Bendtsen 2000). This means that whatever causes the lower pain threshold in some people may also cause them to have chronic headaches.

Migraine Headaches

Migraines usually first begin between the ages of ten and thirty-five and decrease after age fifty. Frequency varies greatly, from infrequent to several times per month. Approximately one in ten people get migraines, and about 75 percent are women (American Medical Association 1989). Some women experience symptoms just before or during their period (menses), indicating a hormonal role.

Symptoms of Migraine Headaches

A migraine headache is characterized by throbbing, pounding, or pulsating pain that lasts from hours to several days. Intensity of pain alone is not a symptom of a migraine, since tension headaches can be as painful or even more painful than migraines, and some migraines may not even have headache pain as a symptom. In some people, the pain may not be pulsating or it may vary in quality. Migraine pain is often only on one side, but it may occur on both sides or move from side to side. Pain can be intensified by movement, coughing, straining, or lowering your head.

Migraines are usually accompanied by one or more of the following symptoms: nausea, vomiting, depression, disturbed sleep, tenderness in the neck and scalp, cold and sweaty hands and feet, and/or sensitivity to light, sound, and smells. A migraine is sometimes accompanied by diarrhea, urinary frequency, fever, chills, facial swelling, irritability, and fatigue. A migraine may be preceded by mental fuzziness, mood changes, and a unusual retention of fluids.

Migraines may be accompanied by an aura, but most often are not. A migraine without an aura is called a common migraine. When present, auras are usually visual and precede the migraine by ten to thirty minutes. People often liken it to looking through a kaleidoscope, with zigzag lines, bright shimmering lights, wavy images, or hallucinations. They may experience blurred vision, eye pain, or temporary vision loss or blind spots. Auras may also be nonvisual, consisting of dizziness, vertigo, speech or language abnormalities, weakness of movement, or tingling or numbness of the face, tongue, or extremities. An aura may occur only on one side even when headache pain is located on both sides, or it may be on the opposite side of a one-sided headache.

Symptoms of migraines are usually incapacitating, and people often feel weak, tired, and sometimes nauseated after the migraine has subsided. People with frequent migraines are more likely to have tension headaches between migraine attacks than those with infrequent migraines.

Causes of Migraine Headaches

Though there are theories about the causes of migraines, the mechanism is still unknown. Most studies have attempted to explain migraines in terms of one particular causative factor and have failed to provide an explanation for the complexity of the symptoms and clinical observations. It's likely that a combination of factors provide input in varying proportional degrees and result in a particular set of symptoms for *any* type of headache. These input factors are trigger points in muscles, emotional stimuli triggering the limbic system (part of the brain) to increase muscle contractions, and substances (including biochemicals such as serotonin and other neurotransmitters) that affect the blood vessels and other tissues in the brain (*vascular system input*), causing them to become inflamed and swollen, and result in a headache.

It is theorized that the sum of the vascular system input plus the input from trigger points and emotional stimuli determines whether or not pain is a symptom, and if so, how intense the pain is. This could explain how some people can have trigger points or experience emotional duress without having headaches or migraines, while others get severe headaches. People who tend to have migraines and tension headaches that occur at the same time are likely to have a very strong input from emotional factors, or possibly abuse drugs (Olesen 1991).

Triggers of Migraine Headaches

Known triggers of migraines include alcohol, smoking or exposure to smoke, weather changes, allergies, altitude changes, jet lag, hormonal changes, stress, sun glare, flashing lights, constipation, some medications, birth control pills, hormone replacement drugs, strong smells such as petroleum fumes and perfumes or colognes, and foods that contain caffeine, monosodium glutamate (MSG), and nitrates (processed meats, bacon, and hot dogs). Insufficient food, water, sleep, or exercise can also cause migraines.

Trigger Points and Migraine Headaches

One study demonstrated that trigger points may play a far greater role in the perpetuation of migraines than previously thought (Calandre et al. 2006). The study compared patients at a headache clinic who suffered from frequent migraines with both nonclinic subjects with fewer migraine attacks and healthy control subjects who, at most, had infrequent tension headaches. The researchers examined specific muscles for trigger points and found that 93.9 percent of the migraine subjects had trigger points with referred pain patterns that reproduced their migraine pain and other symptoms. By comparison, only 29 percent of the healthy subjects had pain referred to the same areas, and the pain was not migrainelike in quality. Pressing the trigger points of migraine subjects could reproduce the location of pain, the throbbing quality, light and sound sensitivity, and other symptoms that were common for that person. In 30.6 percent of migraine subjects, pressing muscles with trigger points actually caused a full-blown migraine that required immediate treatment.

The researchers discovered that the longer the history of migraines and the more frequent the attacks, the greater the number of trigger points the person had in their muscles. About 74 percent of the trigger points were found in the temporalis and suboccipital muscles. Other trigger points were usually only found in additional muscles when the subject had more than four trigger points and the condition had been going on for some time. This means that the longer the migraines and trigger points are left untreated, the greater number of trigger points that will form and the more migraines you will get—a self-perpetuating cycle. (Note: For some reason this study didn't include checking the sternocleidomastoid muscle for trigger points, which would have revealed an even higher rate of correlation between trigger points and migraines and headaches. Also, the sternocleidomastoid would likely have been one of the muscles in which trigger points were more frequently found.)

Trigger points can cause many symptoms other than referred pain, such as dizziness, vertigo, diarrhea, painful periods, colic, heart palpitations, and other conditions. Knowing this, the researchers theorized that the trigger points themselves could be responsible for the changes in the nerves and blood vessels in the brain, rather than the vascular system necessarily being a separate and distinct input system on its own. Their theory makes sense, given that palpation of trigger points can reproduce nonpain migraine symptoms and even evoke a migraine, that treating trigger points can prevent or stop a migraine if treatment is done early enough, and that a greater number of trigger points correlates to greater frequency of migraines and length of the condition.

So which came first? Did the trigger points in certain muscles lead to the development of migraines and then a self-perpetuating cycle began, or did the migraines come first and lead to development of an increasing number of trigger points? In any case, this discovery is very heartening, as it means treating trigger points can have a significant impact on reducing or eliminating migraines.

Other Types of Migraines

There are a few types of migraines that won't likely be helped by trigger point self-help techniques, but even in these cases it would still be wise to read through the section on perpetuating factors and eliminate any factors that might apply. A *headache-free* migraine has an aura but no pain. An *ophthalmoplegic* migraine begins in the eye and is accompanied by vomiting, drooping eyelids, and paralysis of the nerves responsible for eye movement. *Basilar artery* migraine, which affects mostly young people, is characterized by a severe headache, vertigo, double vision, slurred speech, and lack of muscle coordination. *Carotidynia*, more common in older people, produces a deep pain that is either dull and aching or piercing in the jaw or neck, and usually tenderness and swelling over the carotid artery in the neck. A *status* migraine is a rare type characterized by intense pain that lasts more than seventy-two hours and may lead to hospitalization.

Cluster Headaches

Cluster headaches primarily affect men between twenty and forty years old. They come on suddenly and are severe, and occur for a series of days, weeks, or months and then disappear. They may recur seasonally or randomly.

Symptoms of Cluster Headaches

Onset occurs most frequently within two to three hours of falling asleep, during a REM phase of sleep, when dreaming occurs. The pain is typically steady and feels like a sharp, burning, or boring pain on one side of the head or in and around one eye, but it can involve a whole side of the face from the neck to the temples. The pain quickly gets worse, peaking within five to ten minutes, with the peak pain lasting from thirty minutes to two hours. It may be accompanied by a red, flushed face. A runny nose, nasal congestion, swelling under or around the eye, or a red or teary eye with a small pupil may occur, usually on the same side as the headache.

Causes and Triggers of Cluster Headaches

Alcohol, tobacco, and drugs that dilate or constrict blood vessels are known to trigger cluster headaches, suggesting that changes in the walls of blood vessels of the head and/or around the eye area may be at least partially responsible. This may be due to a sudden release of histamine or serotonin by body tissues (histamine is released in response to allergies, but there may be other triggers as well).

One research team found that 81 percent of patients with cluster headaches also had sleep apnea, a condition where the person stops breathing for ten seconds or longer while sleeping (Graff-Radford and Newman 2004). This may explain why treatment with oxygen relieves cluster headaches for some people, particularly if the headaches tend to occur at night. People are generally unaware that they suffer from sleep apnea. Symptoms include excessive sleepiness during the day, difficulty concentrating, and poor memory. If you suffer from cluster headaches, you should be evaluated for sleeping disorders.

Note that the triggers and causes of cluster headaches are the same as some of the triggers and causes of migraines, and of trigger points. Oxygen deprivation of muscle cells plays a role in causing cluster headaches, and it also activates trigger points. Though the role of trigger points in activating and perpetuating cluster headaches has not yet been studied, treating trigger points and eliminating perpetuating factors will likely help resolve cluster headaches.

Headaches from Trauma

Neck injuries are the most common cause of post-traumatic headaches. In a study of patients following rear-end motor accidents, 62 percent of people reported feeling neck pain within six to seventy-two hours, and of those, 82 percent also reported headache symptoms. Twelve weeks after the accident, 73 percent still had headaches (Packard 2002). Even accidents that may seem minor at the time may cause significant damage; in fact, there is little correlation between the damage to the vehicles or the speeds involved in the accident and the amount of injuries to soft tissue and the cervical spine. Slip and fall injuries can cause damage similar to whiplash. Whiplash injuries can lead to TMJ dysfunction, affecting the muscles in the face and causing headaches due to referred pain.

Injuries can cause long-term damage and ongoing problems. Because injured tissues are repaired with dense connective scar tissue, they lack the strength and elasticity of the original, normal tissue. The damaged area is easily reinjured due to weakness and limited range of motion, and the muscle is also more easily fatigued. Damage to muscles, ligaments, joint capsules, and other tissues in the neck, including the sternocleidomastoid and scalene muscles, can lead to central sensitization and thus to chronic headaches (Packard 2002).

Though symptoms from whiplash injuries generally improve over a period of weeks or months, up to 40 percent of people have symptoms that last for more than six months and a small percent become disabled (Packard 2002). Often symptoms disappear after a short time, then recur later. For this reason, I encourage people to wait several months before signing insurance release forms, to make sure the full extent of injuries is known while medical payments for diagnosis and treatment are still available.

It is important for both the patient and the practitioner to recognize that some loss of function is inevitable after a significant injury. However, it's still likely that you can obtain significant relief from a combination of various therapies. Self-treatment of trigger points can play a big role in reducing pain and restoring function.

Secondary Headaches

A headache resulting from a known underlying condition is referred to as a *secondary headache*. It may be due to cerebrovascular disease, a tumor, a blow to the head, an infection, diabetes, thyroid disease, or tooth, eye, or ear problems—or some other primary condition. Medications can also cause secondary headaches. If you're taking medications, ask your pharmacist if that is a possibility. Treatment of secondary headaches is aimed at addressing the primary condition, but treatment of trigger points may still help with the associated headaches.

Some headaches are triggered by coughing, exercise, orgasms, or exposure to cold temperatures or high altitudes. Because these headaches are usually short in duration and infrequent, they rarely lead to development of trigger points, so they aren't addressed in this book. Treatment is usually aimed at minimizing or eliminating the cause.

Great News: Treating Trigger Points Can Help!

Studies have shown that people who have headaches are almost twice as likely as healthy control subjects to have postural abnormalities, including head-forward posture, and to have trigger points in the back of the neck, particularly in the suboccipital muscles (discussed in chapter 11). Interestingly, people with migraines were shown to have the same prevalence of postural abnormalities and number and location of trigger points as people with tension headaches, even when they tend to have one-sided migraines (Marcus et al. 1999).

People who suffer from both migraines and tension-type headaches are far more likely to have a greater number of active trigger points (Marcus et al. 1999). The greater the number of active trigger points, the more frequent and severe the headaches. With one-sided headaches, a greater number of active trigger points are located on the same side as the headache. Trigger points will be more tender during a headache and will probably be more tender just prior to and immediately after the headache.

This means that the probability of trigger points being part or all of the problem in the majority of headaches is likely to be high, and there are estimates that the majority of headaches are due at least in part to trigger points (Simons, Travell, and Simons 1999). So the great news is that you can probably relieve much or all of your headache pain with a combination of trigger point self-treatments and identifying and eliminating all the perpetuating factors to the extent possible.

Treating Headaches with Trigger Point Therapy

If you have headaches, you are likely to have trigger points in your neck and head muscles that, when pressed, will refer pain to the areas where you normally feel your headaches. These areas will likely be tender, too. The intensity of your headaches will correlate with the intensity of the tenderness of the muscles causing the referred pain. In all likelihood, trigger points in more than one muscle of the neck and head are causing overlapping referral patterns, so you need to locate all of the trigger points involved for lasting relief.

It is important to treat trigger points when you don't have a headache. You will still be able to identify the trigger points, and treatments should help prevent the onset of a headache in the first place. Don't wait until you start to feel preliminary headache symptoms; you won't feel like moving once a severe migraine or other bad headache starts to manifest, let alone go to an appointment. Plus, the increased tenderness of the muscles during a headache will make treatments less tolerable.

Most people make the mistake of discontinuing treatments when their symptoms have subsided to a low level. This is too soon. Ideally, all of your symptoms should be entirely eliminated and you should experience a symptom-free period before you stop regular self-treatments or appointments with a practitioner. And if your symptoms start to return, don't wait until they get intolerable before you start treatment again. Your condition will just get more complicated again and require a longer treatment period. If you do decide to see a practitioner, at the first visit schedule all of your appointments for the first six weeks. At the end of six weeks, your practitioner can make a recommendation for the next six weeks.

Headache Medications: To Take, or Not to Take?

The decision whether to take medications for headaches is one you should consider carefully. As mentioned in chapter 2, taking analgesics early on can be useful, as it may help you short-circuit the pain cycle. However, complications may occur from side effects of headache medications, including *rebound effects*, meaning that the headache may go away at the time, but the medication will predispose you to getting headaches that are even more frequent and intense. Anyone who uses headache medications more than one or two days a week, even over-the-counter pain relievers, may be suffering from rebound and should consult a doctor.

If you do choose to take medication for your headaches, see your health care provider if you experience any unusual symptoms, including irregular heartbeat, depression, fatigue, extreme sleepiness, nausea, vomiting, diarrhea, constipation, stomach pain or cramps, dry mouth, extreme thirst, changes in skin color, or a cough that won't go away.

Conclusion

In this chapter you have learned about the most common types of headaches and their symptoms and causes. The longer you've been experiencing headaches and the more intense the pain, the greater the likelihood that central sensitization and trigger points are keeping your headache cycle going, even if the initial instigating factors are no longer present. A combination of trigger points and perpetuating factors is probably involved in causing and perpetuating your headaches, which means that by treating both, you are likely to get a great deal of relief from your headaches, and hopefully complete relief. Treat your trigger points when you don't have a headache. This will help prevent headaches from starting in the first place. Don't discontinue treatments until after you have a headache-free period.

The next chapter will discuss the temporomandibular joint and how problems with both the joint and trigger points in the muscles around the mouth can contribute to headaches.

Chapter 4

Temporomandibular Joint (TMJ) Dysfunction

In the previous chapter, you learned that people with temporomandibular disorders are twice as likely to get headaches as people without TMD, and that their headaches are more frequent and severe (Kemper and Okeson 1983). You also learned that headaches are the most common symptom in people with TMJ problems, usually a tension-type headache but sometimes a combination of migraines and tension headaches. Even if you are not aware of having TMJ problems, trigger points in your face and in and around your mouth may be contributing to your headaches to one degree or another. This chapter will help you evaluate whether TMD is an important factor for you, and whether you should seek help from a dentist.

The Temporomandibular Joint

The temporomandibular joint is different from other joints. The joint is surrounded by dense, fibrous connective tissue that doesn't have blood vessels in it, and the disk inside the joint is composed of the same type of tissue. This unique type of tissue is capable of changing shape, or "remodeling" itself in response to physiological stresses on the joint. This is beneficial to a point, as it allows the TMJ to adapt to minor changes in your bite. However, once the disk has disintegrated due to long-term damage, it can no longer regenerate tissue and is gone permanently.

Symptoms and Causes of TMJ Dysfunction and Trigger Points

Temporomandibular joint dysfunction can be divided into two categories: problems in the joint itself due to alignment problems and inflammation, and untreated trigger points in the muscles in and around your mouth. Often these components occur in combination, and trigger points can eventually lead to changes in the joint or to *malocclusion*, which means that the teeth in the upper and lower jaws don't fit together properly.

People without jaw restrictions can get at least two knuckles (vertically) between their top and bottom front teeth. If you can't do this, you don't have a normal range of motion. If your jaw deviates to one side when you open your mouth, the side it deviates toward is the one more likely to contain trigger points. If you experience a great deal of pain when you press right over the joint and inside your ear, the joint itself is probably inflamed.

Some disorders affecting the TMJ restrict range of motion or cause noises such as clicking but are relatively painless. Clicking occurs when the disk is not tracking in the joint properly, and because of the joint's capacity to remodel itself, the disk will eventually change shape, which may lead to a locking jaw and possibly pain. Inflammation and osteoarthritis may accompany changes in the joint. Latent trigger points may cause symptoms other than pain, so it is wise to treat the likely trigger points even if you aren't experiencing the pain of active trigger points.

Trigger points can be caused by clenching your teeth or grinding them, pressing your tongue against your teeth or the roof of your mouth, abnormal head and neck postures, or direct trauma to the face. People can often remember a specific event that initiated the TMJ dysfunction, such as eating hard food, yawning widely, a whiplash injury, a blow to the face, or a dental treatment, such as the removal of wisdom teeth or wearing braces.

Self-Help for TMJ Dysfunction

You can easily work on trigger points in your face, neck, and head yourself. (Part III will provide all the details for doing so.) If you see a professional, they will want to differentiate between TMJ pain caused exclusively by joint problems, myofascial pain due to trigger points alone, and trigger points perpetuated by joint dysfunction. If you work on your own trigger points, it will likely make it easier for a professional to distinguish between joint disorders and trigger point pain, and your self-treatment may help relieve the joint dysfunction. Because of the possibility of permanent damage to the disk from long-term malalignment problems, it is advisable to treat TMJ-related trigger points as early as possible.

As you work on your trigger points, your bite may change. So if you use a bite guard or are considering getting one, you may want to wait until several weeks into your trigger point therapy; otherwise you may have to be refitted for a new one fairly soon. While bite guards and splints will not prevent you from clenching, they will help protect your teeth and relieve some of the muscular fatigue. The soft plastic bite splints available over the counter in pharmacies are too soft and won't help temporomandibular joint dysfunction. You need to be fitted by your dentist for a hard, acrylic bite guard.

Even if your pain is located primarily in your face, it is important to check for trigger points in all of the muscles of your face, head, and neck, since you're likely to have referred pain to your face from one of these muscles. Make sure you supplement with calcium, magnesium, and folic acid, as a deficiency can play a role in grinding your teeth (bruxism). (You'll find more details on calcium, magnesium, and other helpful supplements in chapter 6, Diet.) All of the stretching exercises in part III will be very helpful. Do them regularly unless you experience a painful click or your jaw is locking or dislocates. Stop chewing gum or anything else that requires prolonged chewing. If possible, consult with a practitioner who specializes in TMJ disorders.

Pay attention to your posture, especially where you hold your head in relation to your trunk (discussed under "Head-Forward Posture" in chapter 5). The associated strain of head-forward posture on the shoulder and neck muscles causes the jaw to retract, leading to malalignment of the teeth and the temporomandibular joint, in turn leading to the development of trigger points in the chewing muscles, which can eventually cause headaches.

Conclusion

If you don't have a normal range of motion in your jaw, if your jaw deviates to one side when you open your mouth, or if you have pain or clicking noises when you open and close your jaw, you probably have trigger points in at least some of the surrounding muscles. Trigger points can be caused by clenching your jaw, direct trauma to the face, or abnormal positioning of the head, neck, or tongue. Fortunately, the trigger points involved are easy to self-treat, and it's advisable to do so for at least a few weeks before being fitted for a bite guard or having any major dental intervention that could be permanent, since trigger point therapy may relieve all or some of your symptoms or change your bite alignment.

The next part of the book lists common factors that cause trigger points and keep them activated. It will help you figure out why you have developed trigger points and offer suggestions for dealing with these perpetuating factors.

Part II

WHAT CAUSES TRIGGER POINTS AND KEEPS THEM GOING— PERPETUATING FACTORS

If we treat myofascial pain syndromes without . . . correcting the multiple perpetuating factors, the patient is doomed to endless cycles of treatment and relapse. . . . Usually, one stress activates the [trigger point], then other factors perpetuate it. In some patients, these perpetuating factors are so important that their elimination results in complete relief of the pain without any local treatment.

—Doctors Janet Travell and David G. Simons (1983, 103)

Applying pressure to trigger points will probably relieve pain and other symptoms either temporarily or for the long term; however, it won't resolve the underlying perpetuating factors. If you get temporary relief from trigger point therapy but your symptoms quickly recur, then trigger points are definitely a factor, but you'll need to address perpetuating factors to gain more lasting relief. This is particularly important if you have migraines, since a greater variety of perpetuating factors play a role in migraines, and they play a larger role, too.

This section outlines some general causes that activate or perpetuate trigger points and offers many suggestions on how to address the perpetuating factors to help you eliminate headache and TMJ pain caused by trigger points in the muscles of the neck, upper back, and head. (In part III, the chapters on specific muscles will give you suggestions specific to each muscle.) I recommend you read the entire chapter on perpetuating factors since multiple factors are often involved, and up to this point you may not have been aware that these factors could be contributing to your headaches. Because many different factors may be involved in your situation, at the outset you may find it difficult to identify the exact causes of your headaches. But as you begin to eliminate likely causes, and the frequency of your headaches decreases, you'll be able to pinpoint which remaining perpetuating factors are relevant to your situation.

Common perpetuating factors include mechanical stress, injuries, spinal misalignments, nutrient deficiencies, poor dietary habits, food allergies, emotional factors, sleep problems, acute or chronic infections, hormonal imbalances, and organ dysfunction and disease. Laboratory tests that can help you confirm or rule out particular factors are outlined at the end of chapter 7.

As you address perpetuating factors, pace yourself so that the process isn't too overwhelming; try to make it enjoyable. Work on your perpetuating factors over time. You probably can't make all the needed changes at once. An important first step is to start keeping a headache diary so that you can determine which perpetuating factors apply to you. As you begin to address your perpetuating factors, go ahead and start on the self-help techniques in part III.

Keeping a Headache Diary

To help figure out which perpetuating factors are keeping your trigger points and headaches activated, keep a headache diary. Whenever you have a headache, keep track of all of the following information:

- The date and time the headache started

- Where you feel pain (including in your neck and back)

- Intensity of pain: mild, moderate, severe, or very severe

- What you were doing at the time: for example, exercising, working, reading, or lying down

- How well and how long you slept the previous night

- What you ate, drank, smelled, and heard in the twenty-four hours before the headache

- What you were feeling prior to onset of the headache: for example, anger, fear, sadness, stress, joy, or depression

- Any other symptoms

- Anything that made you feel better

- Anything that made you feel worse

- For women, where you are in your menstrual cycle and any hormones you're taking

Make a chart that helps you keep track of this information, or visit my website, www.trigger pointrelief.com, for a sample chart you can modify for your own use.

Chapter 5

Body Mechanics

How you sit, stand, walk, sleep, move, and generally treat your muscles has an enormous effect on the formation and perpetuation of trigger points. Proper posture, furniture that fits and supports you, properly fitting clothing, and modification of certain activities will greatly speed your healing and help provide long-term relief. Learning proper posture, especially head positioning, is critical to treating trigger points since head-forward posture can cause and perpetuate trigger points and be a major factor in headaches and TMJ dysfunction. Reducing visual stress is also important, in part because you may hold your head forward in an effort to see more clearly. Treating new injuries promptly can help prevent the formation of trigger points, and the treatment of older injuries, as well as spinal misalignments and other problems in the skeletal system, can help stop the perpetuation of trigger points.

Mechanical Stressors

Chronic mechanical stressors such as misfitting furniture, abuse of muscles, restrictive clothing, head-forward posture, visual stresses, and skeletal asymmetries cause a self-perpetuating cycle of trigger point aggravation and are among the most common causes and perpetuators of trigger points involved in headaches and TMJ problems. Fortunately, they are nearly always correctable, and minimizing or eliminating them is one of the most important things you can do to break your cycle of headaches.

Misfitting Furniture

Misfitting furniture is a major cause of muscular pain, particularly in the workplace. Sitting at a desk or computer, whether at work or home, places a great deal of stress on your trapezius and neck muscles, but there are many things you can do to minimize this stressor. There are a lot of great gadgets that can help correct your posture, and many of them aren't too expensive, such as lumbar supports, phone headsets, and copy holders. Just sticking a thick catalog under your computer screen to raise it to the proper height can make a big difference. Having these gadgets readily available will ensure you use them as much as possible.

Consider contacting a company that specializes in ergonomics to come to your workplace and assess your office arrangement. They can make some adjustments and help you select furniture that fits your body. Your employer may balk at the cost, but if you end up with health problems as a result of a poor workstation, they'll end up paying for it in lost work time and workers' compensation claims. If your employer won't pay for this, consider paying for it yourself. What is it worth to you to be pain free?

Get Furniture That Fits You

Modifying or replacing misfitting furniture is one of the easiest things you can do to get relief from trigger points, especially those that cause the pain of headaches and TMD. Once it's done, you won't have to do it on a daily or frequent basis as part of your self-help. You'll still need to be aware of your posture, but furniture that corrects some of your counterproductive postural habits without you having to be aware of it is much simpler.

Computer screen. Your computer screen should be directly in front of you, slightly below eye level and slightly tilted back at the top. If you work from hard copy, it should be attached to the side of the screen with a copy holder so that you can look directly forward as much as possible, rather than tipping your head down or turning it too far to the side. You can raise the height of your screen by placing catalogs or books underneath it until it's at the correct level. Evaluate your workstation to make sure that you don't have glare on your screen, that your lighting is adequate, and that your computer screen isn't bothering your eyes.

Keyboard and mouse. Your keyboard and mouse should be kept as close to lap level as possible. An ergonomically correct keyboard and keyboard tray should allow you to keep the keyboard near your lap and use your chair armrests while typing. I see a lot of what I call "mouse injuries": arm and shoulder pain due to using a computer mouse for extended periods of time without proper arm support, which can eventually lead to headaches due to the formation of trigger points in the trapezius and the back of the neck.

Chair. Your elbows and forearms should rest evenly on either your work surface or armrests of the proper height. The armrests must be high enough to support your elbows without you leaning to the side, but not so high as to cause your shoulders to hike up. The upholstery needs to be firm, and casters should be avoided. Your knees should fit under your desk, and your chair needs to be close enough that you can lean against your backrest. A good chair supports both your lumbar area and your midback and has a backrest with a slope slightly back from vertical. The seat should be low enough that your feet rest flat on the floor without compression of your thighs by the front edge of the seat, high enough that not all the pressure is placed on your gluteal area, and slightly hollowed out to accommodate your buttocks.

Other office furniture. If you must bend over reading materials, plans, or blueprints, a tilted work surface will alleviate the mechanical stress on your back and neck muscles to a point, but be sure to take frequent breaks.

Headset. A telephone headset can provide a great deal of relief from headaches, since it will help resolve neck and back pain. Telephone shoulder rests aren't adequate, and if you try to hold the phone in your hand, you'll end up cradling it between your head and shoulder at some point, which is very hard on your neck and trapezius muscles. Get headsets for all of your phones—at work, at home, and for your cell phone.

Lumbar support. A lumbar support helps correct round-shouldered posture. Most chiropractic offices carry lumbar supports of varying thickness. I recommend that you get one for your car and one for your favorite seat at home. Try to avoid sitting on anything without back support, since this causes you to sit with your shoulders and upper back slumped forward. When going to sporting events, picnics, or other places where you won't have back support, bring a Crazy Creek chair or something similar to provide at least some support. You can get one through most major sporting goods suppliers. They only cost about forty dollars—a good investment in your back—and they're very lightweight for carrying. Or consider a lightweight collapsible chair, also available at sporting goods stores.

Bedtime Furniture

You probably spend about one-third of your time in bed, so it is extremely important to make sure your pillows and bed are right for you. Sleeping on a couch or in a chair should definitely be avoided.

Pillows. If your pillow is made from foam rubber or some other springy material that will jiggle your neck, get rid of it! Vibrations from these pillows will aggravate trigger points. (However, memory foam pillows are fine.) Your pillow should support your head at a level that keeps your spine in alignment and is comfortable when you are lying on your side. Chiropractic offices usually carry well-designed pillows. I always take my pillow with me when I travel; that way I know I have something comfortable to sleep on, and it comes in handy if I get stuck in an airport.

Bed. A bed that is too soft can cause a lot of muscular problems. You may not even realize that your bed is too soft. People usually insist their mattress is firm enough, but when queried further they admit that sleeping on a mat on the floor gives them relief when their pain is particularly bad. Try putting a camping mat on the floor and sleeping on it for a week. If you feel better, your mattress isn't firm enough, no matter how much money you spent on it or how well it worked for someone else. Different people need different kinds of mattresses. An all-cotton futon is very firm and may be best for some people. Mattresses really only last about five to seven years, and after that time they should be replaced. Also consider that if your partner is heavier, you may be unaware that you are bracing yourself slightly in order not to roll into them. Some types of mattresses can accommodate couples who need different degrees of firmness.

Abuse of Muscles

Properly fitting furniture won't help as much if you aren't also conscientious about avoiding poor posture. If you slouch at your desk or on your couch or read in bed, your muscles will suffer. Abuse of muscles includes poor body mechanics (such as lifting improperly), long periods of immobility (such as sitting at a desk without a break), repetitive movements (such as keyboarding or using a computer mouse), holding your body in an awkward position for long periods (as in certain professions, such as dentistry and auto repair), and excessively quick and jerky movements (as in certain sports).

Be sure to sit while putting clothing on your lower body. When having a conversation, turn and face the person rather than rotating your head in their direction. Learn to lift properly (using your knees, not your back), and take frequent breaks from anything you must do for long periods of time. If your hearing is impaired, get a hearing aid and wear it; if you can't hear properly, you will constantly turn your head to one side, stressing your trapezius and neck muscles. For women, if your breasts are large enough that they cause backaches, your insurance company may cover breast reduction surgery if your doctor recommends it. However, you should carefully consider the risks of surgery before pursuing this option.

Self-help technique: Take frequent breaks. Any time you must sit for long periods, take frequent breaks. One good trick is to set a timer across the room; you'll have to get up to turn it off.

Self-help technique: Notice when you're tensing … and relax! Notice whether you're hiking your shoulders up or tightening muscles, particularly when you're under stress. Take a minute to mentally assess your body, noticing where you're holding tension. Whenever you come to an area that's tense, take a deep breath and consciously relax the area as you exhale. Do this several times each day. You will need to retrain yourself to break the habit of holding tension in certain areas.

Self-help technique: Increase range of motion *gently.* If you have a habit of immobilizing your muscles to protect against pain, you need to increase your range of motion gently and gradually as you inactivate trigger points. Don't keep stressing the muscle to see if it still hurts or to demonstrate to health care professionals where you have to move it to in order to get it to hurt. If you keep repeating this motion, you will just keep the trigger points activated.

Self-help technique: Stop clenching your jaw. If you clench your jaw or grind your teeth, see a dentist for help. Try taking calcium, magnesium, folic acid, and B complex supplements. Stress-reduction techniques will also help.

Self-help technique: Do tongue rolls. Tongue rolls help relax the muscles of the mouth. First, take three deep breaths through your mouth, and then close your mouth and continue breathing deeply through your nose throughout the rest of the exercise. Keeping your lips sealed, begin rolling your tongue in big circles on the outside of your teeth but inside your lips. Roll your tongue ten times in each direction. If you can't do this many repetitions initially, do as many as are comfortable.

Clothing

You may be surprised to learn that what you wear and how you wear it can cause or perpetuate trigger points. Since constricting clothing can impair circulation, it can directly cause trigger points. Footwear could be involved in headaches indirectly. Any time you're standing or walking, your feet affect your entire posture and gait. High heels and other footwear with heels can cause muscular tension throughout your body, thereby contributing to trigger points. Luckily, clothing is a problem that's easily correctable.

Self-help technique: Loosen your clothing. Constricting clothing can lead to impaired circulation and muscular problems. My rule of thumb is if clothing leaves an elastic mark or indentation on your skin, it is too tight and is cutting off proper circulation. Check your socks, belts, waistbands, bras, and ties to see if they're too tight.

Self-help technique: Carry your purse or daypack properly. If you carry a purse, get one with a long strap and put the strap over your head so that you wear it diagonally across your torso rather than over one shoulder, and keep its contents light. If you use a daypack, put the straps over both shoulders. When you carry a purse or pack over one shoulder, you have to hike up that shoulder at least a little to keep the strap from slipping off, no matter how light your purse or pack may be.

Self-help technique: Choose appropriate footwear. While correcting foot supination (more weight on the inside of your foot) or pronation (more weight on the outside of your foot) is essential for some people, I think almost everyone can benefit from using some kind of foot support inserted in their shoes. Shoes rarely have adequate arch support, and this affects muscles all the way up through your body. My favorite noncorrective orthotics are the Superfeet brand. They have a deep heel cup, which helps prevent pronation and supination, and they provide excellent arch support. Superfeet has a variety of models, including cheaper, noncustom trim-to-fit insoles and moderately priced custom-molded insoles. Their products can provide support in a wide variety of footwear. Visit www.superfeet.com to learn more about their products. If you find you need corrective orthotics, you will need to see a podiatrist. As noted above, don't wear high heels, cowboy boots, or other shoes with heels.

Head-Forward Posture

Head-forward posture leads to the development and perpetuation of trigger points and also plays a big role in both migraine and tension headaches. Have someone look at your side profile to see if your head is farther forward than your trunk. The farther you hold your head forward of your shoulders, the more trigger points you're likely to develop, and the more frequent your headaches are likely to be (Marcus et al. 1999). Postural exercises can help eliminate head-forward posture.

Self-help technique: Use lumbar support. Poor posture while sitting, whether in a car, at a desk, in front of a computer, or while eating dinner or watching TV, can cause or aggravate head-forward posture. Using a good lumbar support everywhere you sit will help correct poor sitting posture and, ultimately, head-forward posture.

Self-help technique: Do postural exercises. To develop proper posture and reduce head-forward posture, stand with your feet about four inches apart, with your arms at your sides and your thumbs pointing forward. Tighten your buttocks to stabilize your lower back, and then, while inhaling, rotate your arms and shoulders out and back (rotating your thumbs backward) and squeeze your shoulder blades closer together behind you. While holding this position, drop your shoulders down and exhale. Move your head back to bring your ears in line with your shoulders, and hold this position for about six seconds while breathing normally. (When moving your head, don't tilt your head up or down or open your mouth.) Relax, but try to maintain good posture once you release the pose. If holding this position feels uncomfortable or stiff, try shifting your weight from your heels to the balls of your feet, which will cause your head to move backward over your shoulders. Repeat this exercise frequently throughout the day to develop good posture. Do it every hour or two. It is better to do one repetition six or more times per day than to do six repetitions in a row (Travell and Simons 1983).

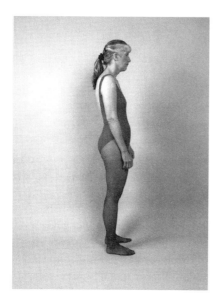 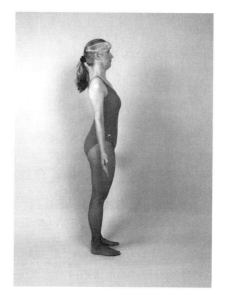

Visual Stress and Trigger Points

Visual stress while doing computer work was found to play a significant role in the development of trigger points, and that role was even greater when combined with postural stresses. One study found that glare, inadequate lighting, poor screen resolution, and flicker (due to low refresh rates) aggravated trigger points (Treaster et al. 2006). The researchers theorized that visual stress increases the level of mental concentration required, and since greater mental concentration has been shown to increase muscle contraction and tension, this could explain how computer work causes or activates trigger points. The study didn't address the effects of vision problems, but it stands to reason that someone who needs to get glasses or needs to have their prescription adjusted would also experience visual stress.

Self-help technique: Adjust your computer screen. Adjust the brightness of your screen and the position of your monitor and seating arrangement so you don't get glare on your screen, while still maintaining an ergonomically correct setup. You may also want to try a nonglare screen cover. The older the monitor, the more likely you will have problems with flicker and glare. You may need to purchase a new monitor. Fortunately, new flat screen monitors are now relatively inexpensive.

Self-help technique: See your eye doctor. If you wear glasses or contacts, make sure your prescription is current. If you wear reading glasses, make sure you can see far enough when you use them. Don't tilt your head down to look through bifocals. If a reflection on your glasses causes you to tilt or tip your head, change your position or the position of the light.

Skeletal Asymmetries

A skeletal asymmetry, including a shorter leg and a small hemipelvis (the part of the pelvis you sit on), can contribute to trigger points involved in headaches. Fortunately, these can be corrected inexpensively and noninvasively with a pad that goes in one shoe or a pad that goes on your chair under one buttock. (In this book, the term "shorter leg" refers to a true leg length inequality, where the bones are actually shorter on one side, rather than the "shorter leg" caused by a spinal misalignment, which is a term chiropractors use when one hip is higher than the other, giving the appearance of one leg being shorter than the other.) Other skeletal disproportions can also be corrected. For example, a long second toe can be corrected with shoe orthotics, and short upper arms can be corrected with ergonomically correct furniture.

Injuries

Injuries are one of the most common initiators of trigger points in general, and they often play a role in the development of chronic headaches and TMJ problems. A healthy muscle is pliable to the touch when not in use but will feel firm if called upon for action. If a muscle feels firm at rest, it is tight in an unhealthy way, even if you work out.

I like to use an analogy of a rubber band and a stick. If a sudden, unexpected force is applied to a stick, it's likely to be damaged, and the same is true of a tight muscle, where the force could be something like a fall or a car accident. If, however, a sudden force is applied to a rubber band, it will stretch to absorb the force instead, and the same is true of a pliable, healthy muscle, making it much less likely to be injured. A muscle may be tight and restricted without you being aware of it, since latent trigger points restrict range of motion to some degree and almost everyone has some latent trigger points. These muscles containing latent trigger points can be injured easily if a sudden force is applied.

New Injuries

As discussed previously, treating an injury when it first occurs can prevent trigger points from forming and help you avoid an escalating pain cycle. See an acupuncturist or massage therapist who is experienced in working with recent injuries. You may also need to see a chiropractor or osteopathic physician.

Self-help technique: Treat new injuries. If you have an injury, begin treatment as soon as possible. Apply cold during the first forty-eight hours, and use some form of arnica homeopathic remedy orally and/or topically as soon as possible. You can get Chinese herb formulas for trauma from an acupuncturist or possibly a health food store. Have these available in your medicine cabinet since it may be hard for you to go to the store after you are injured, and because they work best when you start taking them immediately after the injury.

Surgeries and Scars

A surgery is likely to leave some scar tissue, which can perpetuate trigger points. Scar tissue can be broken up to an extent with vigorous cross-friction massage, a technique in which you rub both of your thumbs in opposing directions back and forth across the scar. However, most people won't work on their own scars vigorously enough due to the pain it causes. You will probably need to see a practitioner for help. Acupuncture can treat scar tissue and help eliminate the pain from trigger points around the area. I recommend using both cross-friction massage and acupuncture, rather than just one or the other.

Spinal Misalignments and Other Spinal Problems

If vertebrae are chronically out of alignment, the stress placed on the muscle due to tightness and pain can cause trigger points to form, particularly in the neck and back. As you've learned, inactivating trigger points in those areas is crucial to reducing or eliminating headaches and TMJ pain. The misalignment is usually caused by tight muscles to begin with, so a combined approach of skeletal adjustments plus massage or acupuncture is probably necessary for lasting relief.

Skeletal adjustments can be performed by a chiropractor or osteopathic physician. They will likely take X-rays at the initial visit to evaluate your spine. If you have already had X-rays taken, bring them with you so you can avoid the additional cost and exposure to radiation involved in duplicating X-rays.

Chronic pain from herniated and bulging disks may also lead to formation of trigger points. Herniated and bulging disks can be very successfully treated with acupuncture (especially plum blossom technique), but if you don't get some relief fairly quickly, you may want to consider surgery. Spinal surgery has gotten so sophisticated that many surgeries are fairly minor procedures that have you back on your feet the next day. If you have *stenosis* (a narrowing of the central spinal cord canal or the holes the nerves come out of), acupuncture will help with pain but not the stenosis, so surgery may be the best option. With any surgery there is a certain amount of risk, so be sure to discuss this with your operating physician and make sure you understand the procedure. If you are still unsure, get a second opinion from another surgeon. Disk problems and stenosis must be confirmed with an MRI. If you have surgery but your pain continues, trigger points are likely to be the culprit, in which case they need to be treated so that you can experience lasting relief. If you still don't get relief, the pain may be due to scar tissue from the surgery compressing a nerve root, something you'll need to confirm with your doctor.

Bone spurs and narrowed disk spaces can also cause chronic pain and lead to the formation of trigger points. But in a random sample of the population, you will find many people with bone spurs and narrowed disk spaces who don't experience pain, and many people who do experience pain but don't have bone spurs or narrowed disk spaces. Don't assume these are causing your problems, even if a practitioner has made this assumption.

I always start with the premise that trigger points are at least part of the problem, if not all of the problem, and treat accordingly. If a patient doesn't get some relief fairly quickly, then I know something else may be going on. At that point, I refer them to someone who can evaluate them with an X-ray or MRI.

Conclusion

To address perpetuating factors related to body mechanics, start with the simple and less expensive changes in your furniture first. Notice how you are holding your body and start retraining yourself to both relax and learn proper posture. Something that may initially seem irrelevant to your situation may lead to a dramatic reduction in the intensity and frequency of your headaches. Next try replacing any furniture where adjustments haven't proved sufficient. If the self-help techniques aren't effective, consult with a health care professional who can help you figure out which self-help approaches are most important for you, or to get fitted for custom corrective devices.

The next chapter will discuss nutrition and other dietary perpetuating factors.

Chapter 6

Diet

What you eat and drink has a great deal to do with the perpetuation of trigger points. Improving your nutrition, drinking enough water, and avoiding certain foods, drinks, and other substances can greatly decrease trigger point aggravation, and therefore also decrease both the intensity and frequency of your headaches.

Nutritional Deficiencies

It is easy and relatively inexpensive to improve your nutrient intake to see if it will decrease your headache symptoms. Doctors Travell and Simons (1983) found that almost half of their patients required treatment for vitamin deficiencies to obtain lasting relief from the pain and dysfunction of trigger points. They believed it was one of the most important perpetuating factors to address. The more deficient in nutrients you are, the more symptoms of all kinds. Even if a blood test shows that you're at the low end of the normal range for a given vitamin or mineral, it's possible that you could need more of it, since your body pulls certain nutrients from your tissues before it allows a decrease in blood levels of those nutrients.

Several factors may lead to nutrient insufficiency, including inadequate intake of a nutrient, impaired nutrient absorption, inadequate nutrient utilization, increased need by the body, nutrients leaving the body too quickly, or nutrients being destroyed within the body too quickly.

What to Take

Even if you have a fairly healthy diet, you may need supplements. In many places, agricultural soils have been depleted of nutrients by too frequent crop rotations and the use of chemical fertilizers, so food doesn't always provide all of the nutrition we require. Most people need to take some kind of multivitamin and multimineral supplement to ensure proper nutrition, especially those who fall into one of the high-risk groups mentioned below.

Don't megadose on supplements unless a doctor has determined your condition warrants it, since taking too much of certain vitamins, such as A, D, E, and folic acid, can actually be detrimental and could cause symptoms similar to deficiencies. You may want to work with a practitioner to develop a personalized supplement program. Some health care professionals can arrange for testing to determine any inadequacies. This is especially important because some people aren't able to absorb certain nutrients and need to take them in megadoses or have them injected. For example, some people can't absorb vitamin B_{12} and need to get intramuscular injections to ensure adequate levels.

The sections below will discuss the nutrients most likely to be involved in the perpetuation of trigger points. If you have other nutritional concerns or would like more information about any of the nutrients discussed here, *Prescription for Nutritional Healing* by James F. Balch, MD, and Phyllis A. Balch, CNC (2000) is an excellent source. It offers information on vitamins, minerals, amino acids, antioxidants, and enzymes, and lists food sources for each. Sections on common disorders list supplements useful for treating each condition.

Self-help technique: Take supplements. Because some vitamins require the presence of other vitamins for optimal absorption or effectiveness, taking a good multivitamin and multimineral supplement helps ensure that the needed combinations are present. Be sure to check the label to make sure there are adequate amounts of minerals in a multivitamin; if not, you may need to take a multimineral too. In addition, you might need to take additional supplements of some of the vitamins and minerals listed below. Doctors Travell and Simons (1983) found that the most important supplements for treating trigger points were the water-soluble vitamins C, B_1, B_6, B_{12}, and folic acid and the minerals calcium, magnesium, iron, and potassium.

When to Take Supplements

Take your vitamins with food, since some nutrients need to bind with substances found in food in order to be absorbed. You may find that it is best to take your vitamins and herbs when you are *not* sick, with the exception of herbs specifically made for fighting illness. Some pathogens can get stronger from some vitamins and herbs, and you could get sicker. (See the section "Acute or Chronic Infections" in chapter 7 for suggestions on how to head off illness.) Once all of your symptoms have abated, you can resume your regular program of supplementation.

Impaired Digestive Function and Nutrient Malabsorption

If your digestive system isn't functioning well, you probably don't have enough enzymes or possibly hydrochloric acid to break down food properly. Symptoms may include any of the following: gas, belching, bloating, acid regurgitation, heartburn, diarrhea, constipation, pencil-thin stools, undigested food in your stools, and weight gain even though you're not eating excessively. Taking digestive enzymes or hydrochloric acid for long periods isn't a good solution for poor digestion, because they can take over some of the natural digestive functions of your body. Instead, you need to repair your body so it can do its job properly. A naturopath, acupuncturist, or herbalist can help you figure out whether you have digestive problems. These professionals can also give you dietary recommendations based on your unique constitution and any health problems, and can prescribe herbs to rebalance your systems.

Although fasting is often recommended as a way to give the digestive system a rest, it's actually hard on the digestive system. If you want to do a cleanse, use herbs and psyllium, but don't stop eating. Another common misconception is that raw foods and whole grains are the healthiest things to eat. For most foods, it's actually better to cook them (not overcook!) to start the chemical breakdown process so your digestive system doesn't have to work as hard. If you have digestive difficulties, white rice and white bread are easier to digest than whole grain products. As your digestive function heals, your practitioner can recommend the appropriate foods for your constitution.

If you have chronic diarrhea, food won't remain in your intestines long enough for nutrients to be adequately absorbed. You will need to identify and eliminate the source of diarrhea. Acupuncture, herbs, and dietary changes can often successfully address this problem.

I've seen many people who have injured their digestive system by taking too many herbs, or herbs that are inappropriate for their health conditions and constitution. Most herbs should be taken only with the advice of a qualified practitioner. An herb that's beneficial for a friend or a family member may not be appropriate for you.

High-Risk Groups

You may be at a higher risk for nutrient deficiency if you are elderly, pregnant or nursing, poor, depressed, or seriously ill, or if you abuse alcohol or other drugs. If you tend to diet by leaving out important food groups or have an eating disorder, you are also likely to have nutrient deficiencies. And in general, many of us eat diets that are neither balanced nor high in nutrition. If you eat a lot of processed foods, be aware that they don't contain as much nutrition as foods that are freshly prepared.

Vegetarianism and Nutrition

When a vegetarian comes into my office and I suggest there may be a link between their headaches and the lack of high-quality protein in their diet, the argument I usually hear is "I've been a vegetarian for twenty years, and the headaches just started ten years ago!" I believe that a lack of high-quality protein causes a progressive problem, and it may take years for some symptoms to show up.

Most people should not be strict vegetarians. The forms of B_6 found in animal sources are more stable and less likely to be damaged or lost during cooking or preserving than the main form found in plants. In addition, vitamin B_{12} is found only in animal proteins, including dairy products. Even brewer's yeast doesn't contain B_{12} unless the yeast is grown on a special substrate that contains vitamin B_{12}.

Self-help technique: Improve your protein intake. If you're vegetarian, at the very least you should eat organic eggs, as they are a source of high-quality protein. Most vegetarians are not very good about combining foods to optimize the balance of amino acids (the constituents of protein) in their diet, and even if they are, many report feeling better within a few months when they add high-quality animal protein back into their diet, even if it is just a few eggs or a piece of fish once per week or a couple times per month.

Vitamins

Adequate intake of vitamin C and the B vitamins is important for resolving trigger points and headaches. The B complex vitamins should be taken together, since they rely on each other for proper absorption and use by your body.

Vitamin C

Vitamin C reduces post-exercise soreness and strengthens the capillaries; when these tiny blood vessels are fragile, you'll bruise easily. (Hint: If you don't remember how you got a bruise, you're probably bruising too easily.) Vitamin C is essential for the formation of collagen (connective tissue) and bones and is required for synthesis of the neurotransmitters norepinephrine and serotonin. It is needed for your body's response to stress, plays an important role in immune system function, and decreases the irritability of trigger points caused by infection. Vitamin C helps with diarrhea due to food allergies, but taking too much can lead to watery diarrhea or nonspecific urethritis.

Initial symptoms of vitamin C deficiency include weakness, lethargy, irritability, vague aching pains in the joints and muscles, easy bruising, and possibly weight loss. With severe deficiency (scurvy), the gums become red and swollen and bleed easily, and the teeth may become loose or fall out; however, this condition is rare in the United States. Vitamin C is likely to be deficient in smokers, alcoholics, older people (the presence of vitamin C in the tissues decreases with age), infants fed primarily on cows' milk (usually between the ages of six and twelve months), people with chronic diarrhea, psychiatric patients, and fad dieters.

Self-help technique: Get enough vitamin C. Good food sources include citrus fruits and fresh juices, raw broccoli, raw brussels sprouts, collard greens, kale, turnip greens, guava, raw sweet peppers, cabbage, and potatoes. It is currently known that vitamin C daily doses above 400 milligrams (mg) are not used by the body, and that taking 1,000 mg daily increases the risk of kidney stones in people with kidney problems, so megadosing with vitamin C is not necessary. Women taking estrogen or oral contraceptives may need 500 mg per day. Do not take vitamin C together with antacids. Since vitamin C is ascorbic acid and the purpose of an antacid is to neutralize acid, antacids will neutralize vitamin C and make it ineffective.

Vitamin B_1

Vitamin B_1 (thiamin) is essential for normal nerve function and the production of energy within muscle cells. Diminished sensitivity to pain and temperature and an inability to detect vibrations are indicators of vitamin B_1 deficiency. You may also experience cramping of your calves at night, slight swelling, constipation, and fatigue. B_1 is needed for the body to produce adequate amounts of thyroid hormones (for more on this topic, see "Organ Dysfunction and Disease" in chapter 7). Abuse of alcohol reduces absorption of vitamin B_1, and liver disease will further reduce absorption. Antacids, the tannins in black tea, or a magnesium deficiency can also prevent the absorption. Because vitamin B_1 is water-soluble, it will be excreted too rapidly if you're taking diuretics or drinking an excessive amount of water. Vitamin B_1 can be destroyed by processing foods, and by heating them to temperatures above 212°F (100°C).

Self-help technique: Get enough vitamin B₁. Good food sources include lean pork, kidney, liver, beef, eggs, fish, beans, nuts, and some whole grain cereals, if the hull and germ are present.

Vitamin B₂

One study showed that taking 400 mg of vitamin B$_2$ (riboflavin) per day may help reduce the frequency and duration of migraines within a couple of months (Schoenen, Jacquy, and Lenaerts 1998). The study indicated that patients taking vitamin B$_2$ had 37 percent fewer migraines after three months, although when they did have migraines, the severity was not substantially reduced. The effect of B$_2$ was first noticed at about one month, and the full benefit was realized after three months. The researchers theorized that since a deficit of vitamin B$_2$ impairs cells' ability to produce energy for the brain and the rest of the body, this may trigger a migraine.

Self-help technique: Get enough vitamin B₂. Good food sources include cheese, egg yolks, fish, legumes, meat, milk, poultry, spinach, whole grains, yogurt, asparagus, avocados, broccoli, brussels sprouts, currants, kelp, green leafy vegetables, mushrooms, molasses, and nuts.

Vitamin B₆

Vitamin B$_6$ (pyridoxine) is important for nerve function, energy metabolism, amino acid metabolism, and synthesis of neurotransmitters, including norepinephrine and serotonin, which strongly influence pain perception. Deficiency of B$_6$ results in anemia, reduced absorption and storage of B$_{12}$, increased excretion of vitamin C, and blocked synthesis of niacin, and can also lead to a hormonal imbalance. Deficiency of B$_6$ will manifest as symptoms of deficiency of one of the other B vitamins, since B$_6$ is needed for all of the others to perform their functions. The need for B$_6$ increases with age and eating a high proportion of protein. Tropical sprue (a malabsorption disease) and alcohol use interfere with the body's uptake of B$_6$. Use of oral contraceptives increases your requirement for B$_6$ and leads to impaired glucose tolerance (a prediabetic condition). This can lead to depression if you don't supplement with B$_6$, particularly if you already have a history of depression. Corticosteroid use, excessive alcohol consumption, pregnancy and lactation, antituberculosis drugs, uremia, and hyperthyroidism also increase the need for B$_6$.

Self-help technique: Get enough vitamin B₆. Good food sources include liver, kidney, chicken (white meat), halibut, tuna, English walnuts, soybean flour, navy beans, bananas, and avocados, but remember that the forms of B$_6$ found in animal sources are less susceptible to loss due to cooking or preserving than the main form found in plants. There is also some amount of B$_6$ present in yeast, lean beef, egg yolks, and whole wheat.

Vitamin B₁₂

Vitamin B$_{12}$ (cyanocobalamin) must be taken together with folic acid in order for the body to form red blood cells and rapidly dividing cells such as those found in the gastrointestinal tract, and for the synthesis of fatty acids used in the formation of parts of certain nerve fibers. B$_{12}$ is also needed for metabolism of both fats and carbohydrates. A deficiency can result in pernicious anemia, a condition that reduces the amount of oxygen available to all of your tissues, including muscles and their trigger points, adding to the cycle of dysfunction and increasing pain. A deficiency of B_{12} may also cause nonspecific depression (depression that isn't temporary and isn't due to a specific event), fatigue, an exaggerated startle reaction to noise or touch, and an increased susceptibility to trigger points. Several drugs may impair the absorption of B_{12}, as can megadoses of vitamin C taken for long periods of time.

Self-help technique: Get enough vitamin B_{12}. Animal products and brewer's yeast grown on a special substrate are the only food sources of vitamin B_{12}. Strict vegetarians must supplement with this vitamin.

Folate

Folate, also known as folic acid when in the synthetic form, is another member of the B complex. A folate deficiency can cause you to be fatigued easily, sleep poorly, or feel discouraged and depressed. It can also cause restless legs syndrome, diffuse muscular pain, diarrhea, or a loss of sensation in your extremities. You may feel cold frequently and have a slightly lower basal body temperature than the normal 98.6°F (37°C). It can also lead to megaloblastic anemia, a condition where the red blood cells are larger than normal, most often due to a deficiency of folate and/or vitamin B_{12}.

Folic acid deficiency is surprisingly common. In the United States, studies have shown that at least 15 percent of Caucasians are deficient, while at least 30 percent of African-Americans and Latinos are deficient. Part of the problem is that 50 to 95 percent of the folate content of foods may be destroyed during processing and preparation, so even if your diet is rich in sources of folate, you may not be receiving the benefit (Travell and Simons 1999).

Folate is converted into its active form in the digestive system, but this conversion is inhibited by peas, beans, and acidic foods, so eat these separately from your folic acid sources. Those at greatest risk for folate deficiency are the elderly and those who have a bowel disorder, are pregnant or lactating, or use drugs and alcohol regularly. Certain medications deplete folic acid, such as anti-inflammatories (including aspirin), diuretics, estrogens (as in birth control pills and estrogen-based hormone replacement therapy), and anticonvulsants.

Self-help technique: Get enough folate. The best food sources are green leafy vegetables, brewer's yeast, organ meat, fruit, and lightly cooked vegetables such as broccoli and asparagus. As with ascorbic acid (vitamin C), don't take folic acid supplements together with antacids. Also, you must have adequate levels of B_{12} in order to absorb folic acid, and supplementing with only one of these can mask a severe deficiency in the other.

Minerals

Calcium, magnesium, potassium, and iron are needed for proper muscle function. Iron is required for transporting oxygen to the muscle fibers. Calcium is essential for releasing acetylcholine at the nerve terminals, and both calcium and magnesium are needed in order for muscle fibers to contract. Potassium is needed to get muscle fibers quickly ready for their next contraction, and a deficiency may cause muscle soreness during exercise or other physical activity. Deficiency of any of these minerals increases the irritability of trigger points. Calcium, magnesium, and potassium should be taken together, because an increase in one can deplete the others.

 Salt is another important mineral. Don't entirely eliminate it from your diet, especially if you sweat. You do need some salt in your diet unless you have been instructed otherwise by your doctor for certain medical conditions. Inadequate levels of sodium, calcium, magnesium, or potassium can lead to muscle cramping.

Calcium

Tums or other antacids can't substitute for calcium supplements because they neutralize stomach acid, which is needed for the uptake of calcium. If you must take an antacid, take your calcium-magnesium supplement several hours before or afterward to maximize your absorption. Vitamin D_3 is needed for calcium uptake. It is especially important to take calcium for at least a few years prior to menopause to help prevent osteoporosis.

Calcium channel blockers prescribed for high blood pressure inhibit the uptake of calcium into the sarcoplasmic reticulum of vascular smooth muscles and cardiac muscles. Since this is probably also true for skeletal muscles, calcium channel blockers are likely to aggravate trigger points and make them more difficult to treat. If you're taking calcium channel blockers, ask your doctor whether you can switch to a different medication. Consider treating the underlying causes of your high blood pressure with acupuncture, dietary changes, exercise, or whatever is appropriate to your particular set of circumstances.

Self-help technique: Get enough calcium. Good food sources include salmon, sardines, other seafood, green leafy vegetables, almonds, asparagus, blackstrap molasses, brewer's yeast, broccoli, cabbage, carob, collard greens, dandelion greens, figs, filberts, kale, kelp, mustard greens, oats, parsley, prunes, sesame seeds, tofu, and turnip greens. Dairy products and whey are also good sources, but they're contraindicated if you have fibromyalgia or a "damp-type condition" as diagnosed by traditional Chinese medicine.

Magnesium

If you eat a healthy diet, you're probably getting enough magnesium; any deficiency is probably due to malabsorption, kidney disease, or fluid and electrolyte loss. Magnesium is depleted after strenuous physical exercise, but reasonable amounts of exercise coupled with an adequate intake of magnesium will improve the efficiency of cellular metabolism and improve your cardiorespiratory performance. Consumption of alcohol, use of diuretics, chronic diarrhea, or consumption of fluoride or high amounts of zinc and vitamin D increase the body's need for magnesium.

Self-help technique: Get enough magnesium. Magnesium is found in most foods, especially meat, fish and other seafood, apples, apricots, avocados, bananas, blackstrap molasses, brewer's yeast, brown rice, figs, garlic, kelp, lima beans, millet, nuts, peaches, black-eyed peas, sesame seeds, tofu, green leafy vegetables, wheat, and whole grains. Dairy products are also good sources, but they're contraindicated if you have fibromyalgia or a "damp-type condition" as diagnosed by traditional Chinese medicine.

Potassium

A diet high in fats, refined sugars, and too much salt causes potassium deficiency, as does the use of laxatives and some diuretics. Diarrhea will also deplete potassium. If you experience urinary frequency, particularly if your urine is clear rather than light yellow, try taking potassium. Frequent urination causes potassium deficiency, and because potassium deficiency may, in turn, cause frequent urination, an escalating cycle can ensue.

Self-help technique: Get enough potassium. Good food sources include fruit (especially bananas and citrus fruits), potatoes, green leafy vegetables, wheat germ, beans, lentils, nuts, dates, and prunes.

Iron

Iron deficiency, which can lead to anemia, is usually caused by excessive blood loss from heavy menses, hemorrhoids, intestinal bleeding, donating blood too often, or ulcers. Iron deficiency can also be caused by a long-term illness, prolonged use of antacids, poor digestion, excessive consumption of coffee or black tea, or the chronic use of NSAIDs (nonsteroidal anti-inflammatory drugs, such as ibuprofen). Early symptoms of iron deficiency include fatigue, reduced endurance, and an inability to stay warm when exposed to a moderately cold environment. Between 9 and 11 percent of menstruating females in the United States are iron deficient, and the worldwide prevalence is about 15 percent (Simons, Travell, and Simons 1999).

If you believe you suffer from an iron deficiency, see your doctor. You shouldn't take iron supplements, other than what is found in a multivitamin or multimineral, because there are health risks associated with taking too much iron. Also, don't take an iron supplement if you have an infection or cancer. The body stores it in order to withhold it from bacteria, and in the case of cancer, it may suppress the cancer-killing function of certain cells.

Self-help technique: Get enough iron—but not too much. Iron is best absorbed with vitamin C. For most people, food sources are adequate for improving iron levels. Good sources include eggs, fish, liver, meat, poultry, green leafy vegetables, whole grains, almonds, avocados, beets, blackstrap molasses, brewer's yeast, dates, egg yolks, kelp, kidney and lima beans, lentils, millet, parsley, peaches, pears, prunes, pumpkin, raisins, sesame seeds, and soybeans. Calcium in milk and other dairy products, or a calcium supplement, can impair absorption of iron, so you should take calcium supplements at a different time than iron supplements.

Water

It's important to drink enough water, as dehydration can cause headaches. Dehydration is especially common among people who take diuretic medications or drink a lot of coffee or other beverages with diuretic qualities. Try drinking a quart of water at the onset of a headache to see if it can help you.

Don't drink distilled water or rainwater, because you need the minerals found in nondistilled water. If you drink bottled water, make sure you know the source of the water to make sure it's not distilled or the minerals otherwise removed. This industry currently isn't regulated, so you may need to do some research on the company.

Self-help technique: Drink enough water. Drink about two quarts of water per day, and more if you have a larger body mass or sweat a lot. Here's a general rule of thumb for people weighing more than 100 pounds: Divide your body weight by two, and drink that number of ounces each day. So if you weigh 140 pounds, you should be drinking 70 ounces. Drink at least one extra quart per day if it is very hot out, and drink extra water during and immediately after a workout. However, too much of a good thing can also be a problem. If you drink excessive amounts of water, you can deplete vitamin B_1 (thiamin) and other water-soluble vitamins. Also, room-temperature water is better than cold; if you drink something cold, your stomach has to expend energy to warm it up, so it taxes your digestive system.

Improper Diet

Eating foods that aggravate trigger points is a common and significant perpetuating factor for most types of headaches. Depending on your constitution, health conditions, and any food allergies, avoiding certain foods can help enormously in relieving your pain.

Plan on avoiding the foods and substances indicated below for at least two months, in conjunction with receiving acupuncture treatments and/or taking herbs and other supplements, in order to determine whether eliminating the specific item is helpful. Many people will stop consuming a food or other substance for just a short while, perhaps only a week, then decide it hasn't made a difference and start consuming those substances again. Or the foods, beverages, or other substances may be so important to them that they'd rather have pain and other medical conditions than give the substances up. Reaching a conclusion after only a short trial period is one way to justify continuing to consume the substance.

Foods and Drinks to Avoid

You may be reluctant to give up a favorite food or beverage. However, I suggest you read this section and consider that the listed items could be at the root of your headaches. Then you can at least make an informed decision about how committed you are to getting rid of your pain.

Caffeine

Caffeine is frequently used in the treatment of headaches. However, this can lead to rebound headaches, meaning it may help at the time, but it will perpetuate the underlying cause and lead to additional headaches.

Caffeine causes a persistent contracture of muscle fibers (sometimes referred to as "caffeine rigor") and increases muscle tension and trigger point irritability, leading to an increase in pain. It causes excessive amounts of calcium to be released from the sarcoplasmic reticulum and interferes with the rebinding of calcium ions by the sarcoplasmic reticulum. Doctors Travell and Simons (1983) found that caffeine in excess of 150 mg daily (more than two eight-ounce cups of regular coffee) would lead to caffeine rigor. I suspect for some people it could be even less. In assessing your daily intake, be sure to count any caffeine in tea, sodas, and other beverages, and in any drugs you may be taking, and remember that espresso and similar drinks have far more concentrated amounts of caffeine.

Alcohol, Tobacco, and Marijuana

In addition to being a trigger for headaches, alcohol also aggravates trigger points by decreasing serum and tissue levels of folate. It increases the body's need for vitamin C while decreasing the body's ability to absorb it. Tobacco also increases the need for vitamin C.

In traditional Chinese medicine, caffeine and alcohol are said to be very "qi stagnating." The ancient concept of qi is not easily translatable into Western medical terminology. It is thought that qi is energy that flows through 14 main "meridians" and connecting vessels that go to all parts of the body. Qi moves the blood and lymph fluids. When the flow of qi is blocked (stagnation), pain and disease result. Based on today's understanding of body processes, some think that qi refers to the biochemical processes in living creatures; the combination of electrical impulses, neurotransmitters, hormones, body fluids, and cellular metabolism that allow us to be living, breathing creatures. As you read in chapter 1, trigger points form when your fluids aren't moving well, cellular metabolism isn't working properly, and neurotransmitters aren't operating normally, which supports that particular concept of qi, and the resulting pain from qi stagnation.

Marijuana is also very stagnating, and it stays in your system for about three months after smoking it. Stagnation is one cause of pain; therefore, using any of these substances will increase your pain level.

Other Foods

Several other specific foods and drinks may aggravate and perpetuate headaches and should be avoided. These include foods that contain tyramine (a derivative of the amino acid tyrosine), particularly red wine, beer, cabbage, aged cheeses, canned or smoked fish, eggplant, potatoes, tomatoes, figs, avocados, bananas, nuts, peanut butter, citrus fruits, onions, dairy products, yeast, and some beans. Other foods to avoid include chocolate, baked goods, anything containing nitrates or MSG, and processed, fermented, pickled, or marinated foods.

Foods and Drinks to Avoid Based on Pain Type

Certain types of pain are aggravated by certain types of food and drink and helped by others. You may have more than one type of pain, and something that is good for one type of pain may be bad for another. If it is problematic for one type of pain, you should eliminate it from your diet, even if it's listed as beneficial under another type of pain. Of course, you should avoid any food you're allergic to, even if it is listed as a helpful food.

Simply eliminating the foods listed below may not be enough if the underlying condition that was caused by the food is still present. For example, if you've been eating foods that led to the development of fibromyalgia, even if you stop ingesting the food you still have dampness in the muscles that must be eliminated (see Appendix A, A Word About Fibromyalgia). It can be treated with acupuncture, herbs, and the helpful foods listed below.

Qi stagnation. Pain that is sharp and stabbing, worse with stress, and better with activity will be aggravated by coffee and black tea (even decaf!), alcohol, heavy red meats, preservatives, spicy foods, caffeine, sugar, marijuana, and foods that are deep-fried, greasy, or fatty. Pay particular attention to this list if you have migraines, and note that the items on this list are very similar to the foods and beverages discussed in the previous section. Foods that help resolve qi stagnation are beets, chestnuts, dill seed, ginger, oregano, saffron, turmeric, basil, black pepper, chives, eggplant, kohlrabi, peaches, safflower, bay leaf, cabbage, carrots, coconut milk, garlic, leeks, marjoram, rosemary, and scallions. Many people with qi stagnation tend to eat excessive amounts of garlic, cayenne, and other spicy foods because it gives them a rush of energy. Even though it initially circulates the qi, it subsequently stagnates the qi further, making the problem worse.

Dampness. Pain that is achy and worse with damp weather will be aggravated by dairy, pork and other rich meats, roasted peanuts, concentrated juices (especially orange and tomato), cucumber, crab, eggs, tofu, wheat, bread, yeast, beer, bananas, sugar and sweeteners, and saturated fats. Foods that help resolve dampness and phlegm include barley, corn, lemon, mushrooms, garlic, celery, onion, kohlrabi, clams, lettuce, seaweed, grapes, alfalfa, sardines, pears, grapefruit, peppermint, radish, shrimp, almonds, and walnuts. Pay particular attention to this food list if you have headaches accompanied by stuffiness or congestion in your head.

Cold. Pain that is stabbing and worse with cold weather will be aggravated by cold food and drinks and helped by warming foods, such as ginger, cherry, peaches, sweet potatoes, turnips, black pepper, coconut milk, kohlrabi, nutmeg, shrimp, spearmint, cayenne, chicken, garlic, onion, squash, trout, and walnuts.

Heat. If you feel hot and have a pulse faster than eighty beats per minute, a red tongue, and burning pain that feels worse with the application of heat or in hot weather, the pain will likely be aggravated by spicy foods, onion, black pepper, garlic, cayenne, chili peppers, jalapeños, alcohol, and ginger. It will be helpful to eat cooling foods, such as asparagus, bananas, lettuce, salt, wheat, chicken eggs, grapefruit, peppermint, tofu, clams, lemon, potatoes, and watermelon.

Qi deficiency. Pain that is dull and achy, worse with activity, and better with rest will likely be aggravated by dairy, tofu, raw foods and undercooked grains, sweets, hard-to-digest foods, and cold or frozen foods and drinks. Foods that help to fortify the digestive system, such as squash, white rice, ginger, oats, cinnamon, yams, onion, black beans, pine nuts, and small amounts of animal protein, are beneficial.

Food Allergies

Exposure to both environmental and food-related allergens causes the body to release histamines, which perpetuates trigger points and makes them harder to treat. Some people with headaches may experience a great amount of relief if they can minimize exposure to allergens. Avoiding allergenic foods can be challenging when you're dining out, traveling, or eating at someone else's home. Whenever it's feasible, bring along something you can eat so you'll have an alternative.

Self-help technique: Do a self-test for food allergens. There are a few methods for testing for food allergens. One of the best ways is an elimination diet, where you eliminate all suspect foods, then add them back in one at a time, and then rotate foods. You can find instructions for this in *Prescription for Nutritional Healing* (Balch and Balch 2000), under "Allergies." However, most people aren't willing to take this approach, as it requires you to be very disciplined about your diet and keep a careful food diary for a month. As an alternative, *Prescription for Nutritional Healing* offers a quick test. After sitting and relaxing for a few minutes, take your pulse rate for one minute, then eat the food you are testing. Keep still for fifteen to twenty minutes and take your pulse again. If your pulse rate has increased more than ten beats per minute, eliminate this food from your diet for one month, then retest. Another option is a blood test for food allergens, offered by naturopaths and some other practitioners.

Conclusion

Improving your nutrition, changing your diet, and avoiding detrimental foods, beverages, and inhaled substances will likely take some time, but you can start by taking a multivitamin and multimineral supplement and drinking enough water. As you identify which foods you need to avoid, start replacing them with foods high in the vitamins and minerals discussed in this chapter. Be sure you are getting enough protein. Because low blood sugar is a common trigger for headaches (discussed in the next chapter), try eating a small snack at the onset of a headache. If that helps relieve your symptoms, try eating smaller, more frequent meals.

The next chapter covers the remaining perpetuating factors that are most likely to trigger headaches, including emotional factors, sleep problems, acute and chronic infections, hormonal imbalances, and organ dysfunction and disease.

Chapter 7

Other Perpetuating Factors

Several other factors that can perpetuate trigger points are worth mentioning, since they may play an important role in your headaches and TMJ problems. Emotional factors such as anxiety and depression, sleep problems, acute and chronic infections, hormonal imbalances, and organ function and disease can all be involved in the formation and perpetuation of trigger points. Laboratory tests are required to diagnose some of these conditions, so you'll probably need to work with a doctor to determine whether those factors are involved in your headaches and trigger points.

Emotional Factors

Emotional factors can contribute greatly to causing and perpetuating headaches—and many other health conditions as well. It's important to recognize the role of stress and emotional factors in illness and to address them just as you would any other factor. And while it's encouraging that modern medicine has accepted the role of emotional factors, all too often people are dismissed by their doctors as "just being under stress." The appointment ends and their physical symptoms are neither assessed nor addressed. This is particularly true when it comes to pain and depression. If you're in pain long enough, of course you'll begin to feel fatigued, depressed, and anxious. The converse is also true: If you're depressed, anxious, and fatigued long enough, you'll probably develop pain.

Depression

If you experience an unusual desire to be alone, a loss of interest in your favorite activities, a decrease in job performance, and are neglecting your appearance and hygiene, you may be suffering from more than a mild and temporary situation-dependent depression. Clinical symptoms of depression are insomnia, loss of appetite, weight loss, impotence or decreased libido, blurred vision, a sad mood, thoughts of suicide or death, an inability to concentrate, poor memory, indecision, mumbled speech, and negative reactions to suggestions. There can certainly be other reasons for some of these symptoms, and no single symptom is indicative of depression. It is the number and combination of symptoms that leads to a diagnosis of clinical depression. However, if you are having thoughts of suicide or self-harm for any reason, it is imperative that you seek help immediately.

Depression lowers your pain threshold, increases the amount of pain you feel, and adversely affects your response to trigger point therapy. There are many approaches to treating depression, including counseling, lifestyle changes, and medications. While antidepressants may help with the acute symptoms, many of them have side effects. Plus, some medications can exacerbate the underlying condition causing the symptoms, so a vicious cycle ensues.

Anxiety

If you are extremely anxious, chances are you're holding tension in at least some of your muscles and developing trigger points as a result. You may be clenching your jaw, pressing your tongue against your teeth or the roof of your mouth, or hiking your shoulders up around your neck—all of which are particularly implicated in the development of trigger points that cause headaches. Tension in other areas can also contribute to trigger points and indirectly to headaches: for example, if you are tightening your forearms, abdomen, or gluteal muscles, then your back and neck muscles are affected.

Get Help for Emotional Factors

If you are depressed or anxious, you need to address this in order to speed your recovery from pain. Unfortunately, people suffering from severe depression, anxiety, chronic fatigue, or extreme pain often don't have the energy to participate in their own healing. You may have difficulty summoning the energy to cook healthy foods or even get out of bed, and you may not be able to manage to do even mild forms of exercise, such as walking—the very things that would help you start to feel better. You may have a hard time making it to appointments with a counselor or health care practitioner. If this describes you, you need to do whatever you can to get to the point where you can start taking better care of yourself. This may mean taking homeopathic remedies, receiving acupuncture treatments or counseling, or doing the self-help techniques in this book. You may need to take antidepressants or pain relievers for a while until you feel well enough to start using the above suggestions. Just doing one of these things will help get you started in the right direction and improve your energy and outlook.

One of the things I like most about Oriental medicine and homeopathy is that both assume you can't separate the physical body from the emotions. These systems of healing consider both physical and emotional symptoms in developing a diagnosis, and both types of symptoms are treated simultaneously. With acupuncture, there are no side effects and response is usually rapid. With both homeopathy and herbs, the wrong prescription or dosage can have side effects, just as with Western prescription drugs, so it is important to consult with a trained professional. Detailed recommendations for treating either depression or anxiety are beyond the scope of this book, but many excellent self-help books on the topic are available. Also see the section on the thyroid in "Organ Dysfunction and Disease" later in this chapter, since thyroid problems can be an undiagnosed cause of depression.

Self-help technique: Get enough exercise. Exercise increases levels of serotonin, a neurotransmitter believed to play an important role in many body functions, including mood regulation. Because many migraines may be caused in part by a drop in serotonin, regular mild to moderate exercise can probably prevent some headaches. Walking and deep breathing are great for relieving tension and depression. Even walking ten minutes per day can be extremely beneficial, especially if you can walk outside.

Sleep Problems

Sleep disorders, interrupted sleep, and insufficient sleep can all perpetuate trigger points, and both the trigger points themselves and the lack of sleep can contribute to headache pain. The first step in solving this problem is to consider whether you had sleep problems before your headaches started. If you did, then the underlying factors responsible for your sleep problems must be addressed.

If pain disturbs you at night, use the self-treatments described in part III to work on your trigger points when you're awakened by pain. Hopefully this will allow you to fall back to sleep once your pain abates. But if you're using a ball for self-treatment, as described in part III, be sure you don't fall asleep on the ball, since doing so will cut off the circulation for too long and make the trigger points worse.

Be sure you aren't sleeping poorly due to being too warm or too cold. Fortunately, this is relatively easy to address. If you have problems falling asleep, try improving your diet, taking supplements, and drinking enough water (but don't drink too much just before bedtime!). Taking a calcium-magnesium supplement before bedtime can be especially helpful. If noise is waking you, try wearing earplugs. My favorite type is Mack's Pillow Soft silicone earplugs. Also try breathing deeply until you fall back to sleep.

Acupuncture and Chinese herbs may be helpful, especially if your mind is overactive, you sleep lightly and wake frequently, you wake up early and can't fall back to sleep, or you have vivid and disturbing dreams, or, for women, if you're menopausal. Computer use or possibly watching TV in the evening can overstimulate the brain and make it hard to fall asleep and sleep restfully. If urinary frequency is disturbing your sleep, try acupuncture, herbs, and increasing your potassium intake.

Caffeine and alcohol will disturb your sleep or make you sleep more lightly. Even if you only drink caffeine in the morning, it can still disrupt your nighttime sleep patterns. If you choose to give up caffeine, you may experience various withdrawal symptoms (including headaches!), and the first few days can be difficult. It will take about two weeks before your energy starts to even out and you feel like you don't need caffeine to get going in the morning.

If you are continually under stress, or if you're pushing yourself too hard and push through fatigue instead of resting or taking a nap, your adrenal glands will excrete excessive amounts of adrenaline, which can interfere with sleep. A naturopathic doctor can administer a saliva test for adrenal function.

Make sure you aren't being exposed to allergens at night. Many people are allergic to dust mites, which live in bedding, among other places. An inexpensive solution is to use soft vinyl covers over your pillows and mattress. If you have a down comforter or pillow, you may be allergic to the feathers even if you aren't exhibiting classic allergy symptoms, such as sneezing and itchy eyes. Or it may be that your mattress is worn out, or that your mattress or pillows are inappropriate for your body. See "Misfitting Furniture" in chapter 5 for more information and recommendations.

Acute or Chronic Infections

Infections are a very prevalent perpetuator of trigger points that cause headaches and TMJ problems, but they're often overlooked. It is extremely important to eliminate or manage infections in order to get relief from pain.

Acute Infections

Try to head off acute illnesses, such as colds and flu, at the first sign in order to avoid perpetuating trigger points. This is particularly important if you have fibromyalgia, sinusitis, asthma, or recurrent infections, since your trigger points will be activated by illness. Getting sick can set you back by months in your treatment and healing.

Self-help technique: Don't get sick. With lifestyle modifications and preventive care, it is possible to reduce your incidence of illness. When you start to get sick, take echinacea, the Chinese herbal formulas Gan Mao Ling or Yin Chiao, and/or homeopathic remedies as appropriate, such as Oscillococcinum for flu. Keep these herbs and remedies on hand at home so you can take them as soon as you notice the first signs of illness. Once you're past the initial stage of illness, which herbs or remedies you need will depend on your particular set of symptoms, so you may need to consult with a practitioner to determine the proper herbs or remedies.

Chronic Infections

Chronic infections such as sinus infections, an abscessed or impacted tooth, urinary tract infections, and herpes simplex (cold sores, genital herpes, or shingles) will perpetuate trigger points, so you need to resolve or manage chronic infections to obtain lasting relief from headaches, and from trigger points in general. With both sinus infections and urinary tract infections, antibiotics often don't kill all of the pathogens, leading to lingering, recurrent infections. However, antibiotics have the advantage of working quickly, so I often recommend combining antibiotics with other treatments, such as acupuncture, herbs, and homeopathic remedies. This will knock the infection out as quickly and completely as possible and prevent it from becoming a chronic problem.

Sinus infections. Any mechanical reasons for sinus infections need to be dealt with if you are to obtain lasting relief. Naturopathic doctors can use a small inflatable balloon to open up the passages. You may need surgical intervention if the blockage is severe enough. Many people report success using a Neti Pot (available at many health food stores) to flush the sinuses with a warm saline solution.

Patients often tell me they have a "sinus headache." If the only symptom you're experiencing is pain over your forehead and/or between your cheek and nose, it's more likely that this is due to referred pain from the sternocleidomastoid muscle (discussed in chapter 12). Never assume you know the underlying cause of a headache based only on the location and severity of your pain (doctors can make this mistake also). Trigger points may be the major cause of the pain, or you may have a more serious underlying problem that should be diagnosed and addressed.

Herpes outbreaks. A variety of supplements, herbs, and pharmaceutical drugs are used to treat recurrent herpes infections, and some will work better than others for you. If you have recurrent outbreaks, you need to figure out what is impairing your immune system, such as allergies or emotional stress. Sometimes a herpes outbreak is the first sign that your body is fighting an acute illness. This can be a signal to you to take the remedies mentioned above.

Dental problems. If you suspect an infected or cracked tooth, you will need to see your dentist for evaluation.

Urinary tract infections. These infections must be dealt with promptly. You can use over-the-counter Western drugs, Chinese herbs, or cranberry extract or juice (don't use sweetened juice), but if your symptoms don't improve right away, you need to see your doctor. Urinary tract infections can turn into life-threatening kidney infections.

Parasitic Infections

The fish tapeworm, giardia, and occasionally amoeba are the parasites most likely to perpetuate trigger points. The fish tapeworm and giardia both scar the lining of the intestines and impair your ability to absorb nutrients, and they also consume vitamin B_{12}. Amoeba can produce toxins that are passed from the intestines into the body. Fish tapeworms can be present in raw fish. Giardia is most often associated with drinking untreated water from streams, but it can also be passed by an infected person who doesn't wash their hands after a bowel movement, particularly if they are preparing food or have some other hand-to-mouth contact.

If you have chronic diarrhea, it is worth testing for parasites. However, such tests can be costly, and different tests are required to rule out different parasites. A cheaper alternative is to treat a suspected parasitic infection with herbs like grapefruit seed extract or pulsatilla (a Chinese herb) and see if your symptoms improve. However, if you have blood in your stools, you should see your doctor immediately to rule out serious conditions.

Many people report feeling much better on an anticandida diet, and in any case it is a pretty healthy way to eat. The basics of the diet are to avoid sugar in all its forms, simple and processed carbohydrates, fermented foods, yeast, mushrooms, and certain cheeses. There are many herbal products on the market for eliminating candida, including grapefruit seed extract, oil of oregano, echinacea, pulsatilla, and a variety of formulas. Since most of these will also kill off your beneficial intestinal flora, you need to use a good multi acidophilus supplement after treatment, as you would after taking any antibiotic.

Hormonal Imbalances

Women are more likely than men to have most types of headaches. Women are also more likely than men to develop trigger points, and I've noticed this is particularly true of menopausal women. Some teenagers (of both sexes) going through puberty also seem to have a tendency to develop trigger points, leading me to believe there is a connection between life-cycle hormonal changes and trigger points. Obviously, you can't stop yourself from going through hormonal changes, but by making sure you are as healthy as possible and addressing other perpetuating factors, you can make those life transitions as smooth as possible and minimize the development or perpetuation of trigger points.

Organ Dysfunction and Disease

Organ dysfunction and disease, such as hypothyroidism, hypometabolism, and hypoglycemia, can cause and perpetuate trigger points. These are among the more challenging perpetuating factors to control or eliminate. For some people, these conditions may cause or contribute to headache pain and TMJ problems.

Thyroid

Both subclinical hypothyroidism (also known as hypometabolism or thyroid inadequacy) and hypothyroidism will cause and perpetuate trigger points. People who have a low-functioning thyroid gland may experience early morning stiffness and pain and weakness of the shoulder girdle. Symptoms of both subclinical hypothyroidism and hypothyroidism include intolerance to cold (and sometimes heat), cold hands and feet, muscle aches and pains (especially with cold, rainy weather), constipation, menstrual problems, weight gain, dry skin, fatigue, and lethargy. Muscles feel rather hard to the touch, and even if people with hypothyroidism take a thyroid supplement, I've noticed they are still somewhat prone to trigger points, probably because it's hard to fine-tune the dosage to the exact amount the person's body would produce if the thyroid gland were healthy.

Some studies report that as many as 17 percent of women and 7 percent of men have subclinical hypothyroidism (Simons, Travell, and Simons 1999). Contrary to the usual symptoms, some people with subclinical hypothyroidism may be thin, nervous, and hyperactive, and in these cases practitioners may not consider the possibility of hypometabolism .

People with low thyroid function may be low in vitamin B_1 (thiamin). Before starting on thyroid medication, try supplementing with B_1 to see if that corrects your thyroid hormone levels. If you are already on thyroid medication and you start taking B_1, you may develop symptoms of hyperthyroidism, in which case your medication dosage must be adjusted. If you are low in B_1 when you start taking thyroid medication, you may develop symptoms of acute B_1 deficiency, which may be misinterpreted as an intolerance to the medication. After the B_1 deficiency is corrected, you will likely tolerate the medication. You need to supplement with B_1 prior to and during thyroid hormone therapy to avoid a deficiency. Total body potassium is low in hypothyroidism and high in hyperthyroidism, so you may need to adjust your potassium intake as well.

Smoking impairs the action of thyroid hormones and will make any related symptoms worse. Several pharmaceutical drugs can also affect thyroid hormone levels, such as lithium, anticonvulsants, glucocorticoid steroids, and drugs that contain iodine. If you've been diagnosed with hypothyroidism and are taking other medications, consult with your doctor or pharmacist to see whether any of your medications could be causing the problem.

Self-help technique: Test your thyroid function at home. A simple home test to check your thyroid function is to measure your basal body temperature. Place a thermometer in your armpit for ten minutes upon waking and before getting out of bed. Normal underarm temperature for men and postmenopausal women is 98°F (36.7°C). For premenopausal women, it's 97.5°F (36.4°C) prior to ovulation and 98.5°F (36.9°C) after ovulation. If your temperature is lower than this, consult with your doctor.

Self-help technique: Get the right tests. Often, doctors initially test only TSH (thyroid stimulating hormone) levels. The results may still be normal if you have subclinical hypothyroidism rather than clinical hypothyroidism. A radioimmunoassay measures levels of two specific thyroid hormones—T3 and T4—and gives a more complete picture of your thyroid function. If you are depressed, insist that your thyroid levels be tested before you start taking antidepressant medication. If thyroid dysfunction is responsible for your depression, correcting it may resolve the depression, allowing you to avoid antidepressants and their many side effects. I've had more than one patient (especially men) whose hypothyroidism was discovered only after they had been medicated with antidepressants for some time.

Hypoglycemia

Hypoglycemia is an abnormally low level of glucose in the blood. This is most often related to diabetes, but there are several other less common possible causes. A hypoglycemic reaction when a meal is delayed (fasting hypoglycemia) usually indicates a problem with the liver, adrenal glands, or pituitary gland. Missing or delaying a meal won't cause hypoglycemia in a healthy person. Onset of hypoglycemia after a meal (reactive hypoglycemia) usually occurs two to three hours after eating a meal rich in carbohydrates and is most likely to occur when you are under a lot of stress. You need to identify the causes and address them if possible.

If you've been diagnosed with hypoglycemia, you probably know the cause and whether it is reactive or fasting hypoglycemia. The important thing to know is that both types cause and perpetuate trigger points, and make trigger points more difficult to treat. Symptoms of both types are sweating, trembling and shakiness, increased heart rate, and anxiety. If allowed to progress, symptoms of severe hypoglycemia can include visual disturbances, restlessness, and impaired speech and thinking. Avoid all caffeine, alcohol, and tobacco (even secondhand smoke). Normally, the liver converts the body's stored carbohydrates into glucose when blood glucose levels drop, and this helps avoid or slow down a hypoglycemic reaction. When you ingest alcohol, caffeine, or tobacco, your liver considers detoxifying your bloodstream the highest priority, and will not put more glucose in the bloodstream until it is done, resulting in a hypoglycemic reaction.

Activation of trigger points in the sternocleidomastoid muscle by a hypoglycemic reaction may lead to dizziness and headaches.

Self-help technique: Eat small, frequent meals. Symptoms of hypoglycemia will be relieved by eating smaller, more frequent meals with fewer carbohydrates, more protein, and some fat. Low blood sugar is a common trigger for headaches, and the lower your blood sugar, the more severe your headache will be. Therefore, eating small, frequent meals may help with your headaches even if you don't have hypoglycemia. If you are waking up with headaches or pain or are having trouble sleeping, eating a small snack or drinking a little juice before you go to bed may help. Also, acupuncture is quite successful in stabilizing blood sugar.

Helpful Laboratory Tests

Laboratory tests may be necessary to help diagnose some of the systemic and nutritional factors involved in perpetuating your trigger points. The information below is included so that you can discuss these tests with your doctor.

With blood chemistry profiles, an elevated erythrocyte sedimentation rate (sed rate) may indicate a chronic bacterial infection, polymyositis, polymyalgia rheumatica, rheumatoid arthritis, or cancer. A decreased erythrocyte count or low hemoglobin points to anemia. A mean corpuscular volume (MCV) of over 92 fL (femtoliters) indicates the likelihood of a deficiency of folate or vitamin B_{12}. Eosinophilia may indicate an allergy or intestinal parasitic infection. An increase in monocytes can indicate low thyroid function, infectious mononucleosis, or an acute viral infection. Increased serum cholesterol can be caused by a problem with low thyroid function, and low serum cholesterol can indicate folate deficiency. High uric acid levels indicate hyperuricemia and possibly gout.

Iron deficiency is detected by checking the serum ferritin level. A fasting blood test is used to diagnose hypoglycemia, and an additional glucose tolerance test or a two-hour postprandial blood glucose test may be used to rule out diabetes. Measurement of sensory nerve conduction velocities can help diagnose diabetic neuropathy. A low serum total calcium suggests a calcium deficiency, but for an accurate assessment of the available calcium, a serum ionized calcium test must be performed. Potassium levels can be checked with a serum potassium test.

Blood tests can determine serum levels of vitamins B_1, B_6, B_{12}, folic acid, and vitamin C. Any values in the lower 25 percent of the normal range, or below normal ranges, indicate that supplementation would be helpful in the treatment of trigger points. Remember, even if serum levels of vitamins and minerals are normal, you may still benefit from supplements, since the body may extract nutrients from tissues to prevent levels in the blood from dropping.

See "Organ Dysfunction and Disease," above, for a discussion of thyroid function tests. A hair analysis can detect mineral deficiencies, as well as high levels of toxic metals. A naturopathic doctor can perform blood tests for food allergies. Stool samples will reveal if parasites are a problem.

Case Studies in Perpetuating Factors

The following case studies are good examples of how eliminating perpetuating factors can make the difference in obtaining lasting relief from headaches. These are not uncommon examples; they represent the rule, rather than the exception.

Rebecca

A man I met at a trade show told me his wife suffered from migraines, and she later came to me for treatment based on his recommendation. She only came a couple of times, and then I didn't hear from her again. A few years later I was at her husband's business and reintroduced myself to him, saying he probably wouldn't remember me. He replied, "Of course I remember you! You gave my wife the best advice anyone has ever given her." I asked what that advice was, and he said, "You told her to drink more water. Since she started doing that, she doesn't have migraines anymore!"

Nancy

A patient who previously lived in another community had one-sided migraines four times per month when living there. When she began seeing me, she was getting them once or twice per month, and they would last anywhere from two hours to a week. She always got one within six hours of the onset of her period, plus some migraines in between her periods. Other than occasional mild PMS, her menses were normal. She said that her migraines were worse with noise, bright light, and sunlight. She only drank about two glasses of water per day and usually skipped breakfast. She drank one cup of coffee per day and used alcohol a couple of times per week. At the end of her first appointment, I recommended that she increase her water intake and eat at least a little for breakfast, even though she wasn't hungry. We talked about coffee and alcohol, but she didn't think they were triggers for her.

Within the first week, she noticed that when she missed a meal she began to feel a migraine come on, but if she ate a little the symptoms would subside. For the next month, she didn't get any migraines during times she normally would have: when under stress and during her menses. During the second month of treatment, after a few weeks of continued stress, lack of sleep, and some dehydration, she did get a bad headache, but she had been headache free for forty days up to that point.

Her treatment plan for the third month and beyond was to have one acupuncture treatment in the week prior to her menses, but due to a death in the family it was three months before I saw her again. At that time, she hadn't gotten a migraine within the last month, in spite of the holidays and her difficult family situation. She came in only sporadically and reported having an occasional migraine, and soon she discontinued treatments for financial reasons. I ran into her again three years later, and she volunteered that her migraines were pretty much gone. I asked what had made a difference, and she said she had stopped drinking coffee and alcohol.

This is a good example of what happens when you decrease or stop treatments too quickly, and how you need to stop consuming potentially problematic foods or beverages for more than a few weeks to determine whether it can make a difference, even if you initially believe that substance is not a problem for you.

Susan

Twenty-two years before she first came to see me, Susan had developed facial and head pain while doing repetitive and demanding physical work. The pain had gotten so bad over the years that she was almost incapacitated at times, and it was ruining her relationships. She lived in a remote community and had to fly to see me at my clinic, so she initially came for a week and saw me four times during that period. During the first visit I recommended she take calcium and magnesium supplements and decrease her tea consumption. I had her start using moist heat on her trapezius, sternocleidomastoid, and face. Her neck and shoulder pain improved after the first appointment, and she reported that the muscles no longer felt like they were spasming.

During the second treatment we talked about her bite alignment, and she noted that she couldn't touch her teeth together properly. I recommended she see a dentist for evaluation. By the third appointment, she had already been able to reduce her pain medications, she was sleeping better, and her bite had improved. She showed substantial improvement in all of her symptoms by the end of the week.

She returned to her community and saw a dentist, who diagnosed her with a sinus infection, gave her antibiotics, and fitted her with a bite guard. Three months later her symptoms started to get worse again, so she saw an ear, nose, and throat specialist, who told her she didn't have a sinus infection, and probably hadn't had one previously. A different dentist refitted her for a new bite guard.

Because her symptoms were debilitating, she tried Botox injections into her trigger points, but that didn't help. Over the course of that year she visited my clinic six times, for one to four treatments each trip, and each time I would teach her more trigger point self-help techniques. She was steadfast about following all of my suggestions and performing the self-help techniques. She kept mentioning she had pain in her teeth, but she had seen both a dentist and an oral surgeon a couple of times each with no relief, so we proceeded under the assumption that her problem was referred pain. With the change in her muscles in and around the mouth due to trigger point treatments, she needed to be refitted a third time for a new bite guard.

Within the year that I treated her, she also went to several specialists and had X-rays taken a couple of times. She was pain-free some of the time and could often control her symptoms with self-help techniques when they did come back, but periodically the pain would return with a vengeance. I didn't hear from her for a couple of years, and then a friend of hers came to see me. I inquired how Susan was doing, and her friend reported that she was pain free. A different dentist had finally discovered that she had a cracked tooth, which either didn't show up on previous X-rays or was missed. Fortunately, she had persisted in seeking diagnosis and treatment and hadn't let anyone convince her it was "all in her head."

Conclusion

Perpetuating factors can play such a significant role in maintaining trigger points and causing headaches that eliminating them may give you complete relief from pain without any additional treatment. And if you don't work to avoid or resolve perpetuating factors to the extent possible, you may not get more than temporary relief from any form of treatment.

Hopefully you've learned enough about your potential perpetuating factors that even if you choose not to resolve them, you'll be making an informed choice about which you value more: relief from your headaches or continuing to do things that make you feel worse, if they are within your power to change. You will have more control over some perpetuating factors than others. For example, you may not be able to control whether you have hypothyroidism, but you can take thyroid hormones and supplements as appropriate and stop smoking. Much or all of your headache pain is probably within your control. What are you willing to do to change your life?

The next section will teach you how to work on your own trigger points, how to stretch properly, how to care for your muscles, and what you should avoid doing so that you don't make yourself feel worse.

Part III

TRIGGER POINT SELF-HELP TECHNIQUES

In this section, you'll learn how to relieve your trigger points with self-help techniques. Chapter 8 provides general guidelines on how to do trigger point self-treatments and what to avoid, as well as some do's and don'ts for stretching and conditioning. Chapter 9 helps you determine which combination of muscles is causing your headaches. Each of the remaining chapters covers a muscle or group of muscles that can contribute to headaches.

In the muscle chapters, anatomical drawings are provided to help you locate where trigger points are most likely located in the muscle, and what the muscle looks like. Symptom lists and photographs showing pain referral patterns, and lists of common causes and perpetuating factors for trigger points, will help you determine whether a given muscle might be causing your pain. These are followed by helpful hints for dealing with those causes. Photographs and written instructions provide guidance on self-treatment of trigger points. Most of the muscle chapters also include stretches and, where appropriate, conditioning exercises. Each muscle chapter will also advise you to check other muscles that may be involved.

Chapter 8

General Guidelines for
Self-Help Techniques

In this chapter you'll learn how to apply pressure to trigger points properly and how to stretch and condition muscles properly. I'll also offer general guidelines on caring for your muscles in order to prevent the reactivation of trigger points.

General Guidelines for Applying Pressure During Self-Treatments

Applying pressure on your own trigger points is generally easy and can give you a great deal of relief within the first few weeks, but you must perform the techniques properly. You can expect gradual improvement over a period of days and weeks. Review the following guidelines frequently in the beginning stages of treatment, and then periodically thereafter to ensure you are performing the techniques properly.

How Not to Perform Self-Treatments

The most important guideline is this: Don't overdo it! Many people think that if some self-treatment feels great, doing it harder, longer, or more often will be even better. But you can actually make yourself worse by doing treatments too frequently or doing them incorrectly.

Don't apply pressure over varicose veins, open wounds, infected areas, herniated or bulging disks, areas affected by phlebitis or thrombophlebitis, or anywhere clots are present or could be present. If you're pregnant, don't apply pressure on your legs.

If your symptoms get worse or you are sore from treatments for more than one day, stop the self-treatments for a few days until your symptoms improve, then resume doing the treatments more gently and less frequently to see if you can tolerate them without feeling worse or sore. Chances are you were using too much pressure or holding the points for too long. Review these guidelines if that is the case. If you're seeing a practitioner, they may be able to help you figure out any problems with how you are doing the self-treatments. And if you are sore from a therapist's work, be sure to tell them this is happening.

How to Work on Trigger Points

The most important technique for treating trigger points, other than eliminating perpetuating factors, is applying pressure. Use a tennis ball, racquetball, golf ball, dog play ball, or baseball, or use your elbow or hand if instructed to do so for particular muscles. When working with balls, use only the weight of your body to give you the pressure. Don't actively press your back or other body parts onto the balls. The muscle you're working on should be as passive as possible. Only use one ball at a time on your back, not one on each side. If you need to work on your muscles during the workday, I recommend getting a Backnobber, available from the Pressure Positive Company (see Resources) and other sources.

Apply pressure for a minimum of eight seconds (less than that may activate trigger points) and a maximum of one minute (to avoid cutting off the circulation for too long, which could aggravate the trigger point). You can count out the time, saying "one one thousand, two one thousand, three one thousand," and so on. Time yourself first to be sure you are actually counting seconds at the correct speed; don't race to eight as fast as possible.

The pressure should be somewhat uncomfortable but hurt in a good way. It shouldn't be so painful that you tense up or hold your breath. If you're using a ball, and the treatment is too painful, move to a softer surface such as a bed, or pad the surface with a pillow or blanket. Alternatively, try using a smaller or softer ball. You can puncture a tennis ball with a corkscrew to make it softer. If the treatment doesn't hurt at all, keep looking for tender spots or try moving to a harder surface. If you're using a ball for treatment but the trigger point is too tender to lie on at all, try putting the ball in a long sock and leaning against the wall. However, I only recommend this if you can't lie on the ball, since leaning against the wall involves using the very muscles you are trying to work on. You may need to use a combination of surfaces depending on the tenderness of different areas. Over time, as your sensitivity decreases and you're able to work the deeper parts of the muscle, you may need to use a ball that's harder or a different size or move to a harder surface. Experiment to find what's effective for you.

If your time is limited, treat one area thoroughly rather than rushing through many areas. If you hurry, you're more likely to aggravate trigger points rather than inactivate them.

If you're using a ball for self-treatment, be careful not to fall asleep on the ball, since doing so will cut off the circulation for too long and make the trigger points worse. When you're fatigued and in pain and suddenly the pain is reduced or gone, it's all too easy to fall asleep on the ball, so don't use this technique in bed unless you're sure that won't happen.

Where to Find Trigger Points

Search the entire muscle for tender points, particularly the points of maximum tenderness, to make sure you find all the potential trigger points. Use the muscle drawings and pictures in the following chapters to make sure you're searching the entire muscle and not just focusing on the most painful spot. Many times a tendon attachment will hurt because the tight muscle is pulling on it, but if you don't work on the entire belly of the muscle, it will keep pulling on the attachment.

If you find trigger points on one side of the body, be sure to work on the same muscles on the other side, but spend more time on the side that's causing your pain. Except for very new one-sided injuries, the same muscle on the opposite side will almost always also be tender with pressure, even if it hasn't started causing symptoms yet. For back muscles, loosening one side but not the other can lead to new problems. And sometimes the muscles on the opposite side are actually causing the symptoms, so it's always worthwhile to work on both sides.

Work in the direction of referral. For example, if your sternocleidomastoid is referring pain to your facial muscles, work on the sternocleidomastoid first, then the facial area.

When working through the pertinent muscles in chapters 10 through 18, be sure to check the other muscles listed under "Also See," since trigger points in one muscle can keep trigger points in other muscles active. For example, if you effectively treat trigger points in your frontalis muscle (one of the face and scalp muscles) but they quickly recur, you need to check the sternocleidomastoid, because it can refer pain to the frontalis and cause trigger points to be reactivated there.

Pressure on a trigger point may reproduce the referred pain pattern, but this doesn't always occur. So if you have reason to suspect that a particular muscle is involved, work on it anyway and see if it helps relieve your headaches and other symptoms.

Frequency of Self-Treatments

Most people should work on their muscles one time per day initially. Pick a time when you'll remember to do your self-treatments—perhaps when you wake up, when you watch television, or when you go to bed—and keep your balls where they'll be handy (just be careful not to fall asleep on a ball!). If you're sore from self-treatments or your practitioner's treatments, skip a day. If you're seeing a practitioner, don't do self-treatments on the same day you have an appointment.

After a few weeks, you can increase your self-treatments to twice per day as long as you're not getting sore. If a particular activity seems to aggravate your trigger points, try doing self-treatments before and after the activity. If you start getting sore or your symptoms get worse, decrease the frequency.

Take your balls with you on trips, since travel frequently aggravates trigger points. You may even want to keep some balls or a Backnobber at work.

Keep working on the muscle until it is no longer tender, even if your active symptoms have disappeared. Just because a trigger point isn't causing referred pain doesn't mean the trigger point is gone. It has probably just become latent, in which case it could easily be reactivated. If you leave your trigger points untreated or stop treatment too soon, it is more likely that the changes to your nervous system will be long-term or permanent, and that the pain will recur more easily. As your symptoms disappear, you may feel less motivated to do treatments or even forget to do them. Try not to let this happen. But if it does, the important thing is that you will know what to do if symptoms return.

General Guidelines for Stretches and Conditioning

It is very important to distinguish between stretching and conditioning exercises. With stretching, you gently lengthen the muscle fibers, whereas with conditioning exercises you're trying to strengthen the muscle. Doctors Travell and Simons (1983) found that active trigger points benefited from stretching but were usually aggravated by conditioning exercises.

Often people start physical therapy and trigger point therapy at the same time, but this may be counterproductive, as physical therapy usually relies heavily on conditioning exercises unless the physical therapist is familiar with trigger points. In my experience, when the two are done concurrently, over half the time the person's condition either doesn't improve or actually gets worse. I often find myself in the awkward position of asking people to *stop* their conditioning exercises until their trigger points are less irritable. Usually you can start doing conditioning exercises after about two weeks of trigger point treatment and self-help work, but if your trigger points are still very irritable, you need to wait until your symptoms improve. Meanwhile, learn the stretching exercises in this book. As long as you follow the guidelines, these do not need to be prescribed by a practitioner.

If you aren't sure whether an assigned activity is a stretch or a conditioning exercise, ask your practitioner. Also be sure to tell your practitioner all the activities, exercises, and stretches you're doing, because some of these could be contributing to activating your trigger points. I won't cover guidelines for conditioning exercises in depth here, since they should be prescribed by a practitioner, who can also give you instructions for performing them safely and effectively.

Things to Avoid When Stretching and Conditioning

Avoid stretching when your muscles are tired or cold, and don't bounce on stretches. Friends may recommend conditioning exercises that worked for them, but you are a different person with a different set of symptoms, and you shouldn't do conditioning exercises prescribed for them, just as you wouldn't take their prescribed medications. If a conditioning exercise or stretch is aggravating your symptoms, stop doing it. Consult with your practitioner to determine why it is bothering you and how you should proceed.

When and How to Do Stretches and Conditioning

Do your stretches *after* treating your trigger points. If you only have time to do one thing, do the self-treatments and skip the stretches. Trigger point inactivation followed by stretching is more effective than trigger point inactivation alone, but stretching without prior inactivation can actually increase trigger point sensitivity (Edwards and Knowles 2003).

Stretch slowly, and only to the point of just getting a gentle stretch. Don't force it. If you stretch muscles too hard or too fast, you can aggravate trigger points. Hold each stretch for thirty to sixty seconds. There will be little benefit after thirty seconds, but stretching for longer won't hurt you. You may repeat the stretch after releasing and breathing. For any type of repetitive exercise, breathe and rest between each repetition of the exercise.

If your stretches or conditioning exercises make you sore for more than one day, try again after the soreness has disappeared and reduce the number of repetitions. If you're still sore two days after the exercise or stretch, you may be doing it incorrectly or it might not be the right stretch for you and needs to be eliminated or changed (Travell and Simons 1983).

General Guidelines for Muscle Care

In addition to inactivating your trigger points and stretching, you need to take good care of your muscles. This will help prevent reactivation of old trigger points and the development of new ones.

Muscle Awareness

After treatments, gently use the muscle in a normal way, using its full range of motion, but avoid strenuous activities for at least one day or until the trigger points aren't so easily aggravated, whichever is longer. Go slowly and be gentle with yourself.

Rest and take frequent breaks from any given activity, and don't sit for too long in one position. Learn to avoid keeping your muscles in prolonged contractions, where you are holding them tense or using them in a sustained way. To increase blood flow and bring oxygen and nutrients to the muscles, they need to alternately constrict and relax, which normal, fairly frequent movement will accomplish. Notice where you hold tension and practice relaxing that area. Avoid cold drafts.

Lift with your knees bent and your back straight, with the object close to your chest. Don't lift something too heavy—ask for help. Never put the maximum load on a muscle. It's too easy to strain your muscles when you do this.

Exercise Programs

Before doing any type of exercise, warm up adequately. Tight, cold muscles are more prone to injury. As always, as with any exercise, avoid positions or activities that aggravate any medical condition. Swimming is generally a good exercise, and bicycling is easier on the body than running, but in both cases you must take care to avoid straining your trapezius and neck muscles. Any bike that allows you to sit more upright, such as a recumbent or stationary bicycle, is preferable to those that require you to lean over the handlebars.

When starting an exercise program, underestimate what you will be able to do, and err on the side of caution. Many people believe in the adage "no pain, no gain" and think that pushing through the pain will make them stronger. But this just aggravates existing problems and makes them harder to treat. Exercise should be comfortable. Alternate running with walking or, when lifting weights, rest between repetitions and use weights that aren't too heavy. If you tend to overdo things, you need to back off on your activities, then add them back in slowly with the guidance of your practitioner. Returning to activities too soon or doing them excessively will quickly erode your progress.

Gradually increase the duration, rate, and effort of any exercises in small increments that don't cause soreness or trigger point activation. Mild to moderate aerobic exercise is good for overall health and for preventing the recurrence of muscular problems. It's also great for reducing stress. People who exercise regularly are less likely to develop trigger points than those who exercise occasionally and overdo it. Just don't overdo it!

Conclusion

In this chapter, you've learned the basics of trigger point self-treatments, along with what to avoid when doing self-treatments. You've also learned some of the basics about how to stretch, and how to take care of your muscles to prevent reactivation of trigger points and the formation of new trigger points. The most important thing to remember is what *not* to do: Don't overdo trigger point treatments, stretching, conditioning, or exercise programs. Review the guidelines in this chapter frequently in the beginning stages of treatment, and then review them periodically thereafter to ensure you are performing the techniques properly.

The next chapter will help you identify which muscles may be causing your headaches and other symptoms. It will also offer guidance on recording your symptoms and tracking your progress.

Chapter 9

Which Muscles Are Causing the Pain?

To figure out which muscles to work on first, look at the Head Pain Map on page 76, then look at the photos of referral patterns in each chapter and try to find those that most closely match your pain pattern. Read the list of symptoms for each muscle. You'll want to start by working on muscles with referral patterns that look familiar and symptoms that seem similar to yours. Eventually, you should read all of the muscle chapters carefully, because other, less obvious trigger points may also play a role in your pain.

Head Pain Map

As just mentioned, the Head Pain Map on page 76 is your starting point for determining which trigger points are involved in your headaches. Find the areas where you feel your pain, then refer to the chapters listed for each to determine which muscles may contain trigger points that are affecting you. You may need to work on all the muscles listed for pain in a particular area if you can't initially figure out which muscles contain the trigger points that are causing your pain, or because trigger points in more than one muscle may be causing your pain. On the Head Pain Map, the muscles associated with each area are listed in order from most to least common for referring pain to that area, but it may be different for you, so be sure to check all of the chapters before assuming the order of priority will be true for you.

You may wish to copy the blank body charts on pages 77 and 78 and draw your symptom pattern on them with a colored marker. Then you can compare them with the pain referral pictures in chapters 10 through 18. Out to the side of each painful area, note your pain intensity on a scale of 1 to 10 and the percent of time you feel pain in that area, for example, 6.5/80%.

I recommend that you fill out a body chart at least a couple of times per week. Date them so you'll be able to keep them in order. This chronological record will come in handy in several ways: It will make it easier to discern which patterns fit your pain referral most closely. It will also help you recognize the factors that cause and perpetuate your symptoms by matching fluctuations in the level and frequency of your pain with the documentation in your headache diary. And finally, it will allow you to track your progress (or lack thereof) and provide a historical record of any injuries. As your condition improves, you may forget how intense your symptoms were originally, and you may think you're not getting any better. The body charts will help prevent this frustration by graphically illustrating any reduction in the overall intensity or frequency of your pain and the extent of the area affected. You'll be able to see that you are improving, even if you have an occasional setback. One note: Not everyone can accurately draw their pain location, in part due to lack of familiarity with anatomy, so take that possibility into consideration and check muscles with adjacent referral patterns just in case your drawing is inaccurate.

Muscle Chapters

Chapters 10 through 18 cover all of the major muscles commonly associated with headache pain. Each chapter contains an anatomical drawing of the muscle or muscles covered in that chapter, with the letter X denoting the most frequent locations of trigger points. Photographs show the most common pain referral areas for each trigger point. The more solid gray overlay area indicates the primary area of referral, which is almost always present, and the stippled area shows the most likely secondary areas of referral, which may or may not be present. The letter X marks spots where trigger points are most commonly found in conjunction with that referral pattern. There may be additional trigger points, so search the entire muscle.

The pain referral photographs in the muscle chapters show only the most common referral patterns; bear in mind that your referral pattern may be somewhat different or even completely different. Also, you may have overlapping referral patterns from trigger points in multiple muscles. These areas may be more extensive than the patterns common for individual muscles, so be sure to search for trigger points in all the muscles that refer pain to that area. Your pain may be more intense in areas where you have overlapping pain referral.

If trigger point treatments seem effective but you only get temporary relief, start looking for muscles that refer pain or other symptoms to the area where you've located and treated trigger points. It may be that other trigger points (primary trigger points) are activating the trigger points you initially worked on (satellite trigger points). You can't resolve satellite trigger points without first addressing the primary trigger points causing them. For example, if you have lower jaw pain and you can get temporary relief by working on the masseter, consider whether referral from trigger points in the upper portion of the trapezius muscle is keeping the masseter trigger points active. In this case, the masseter contains the satellite trigger points, and the trapezius contains the primary trigger points. Each muscle chapter contains a list of other muscles that may also be involved (under "Also See"), but because everyone's body is so different, you may need to look through the referral patterns in all of the muscle chapters to determine which other muscles may be involved in your case.

I occasionally see something I call "reverse referral," where what is normally the area of referral contains trigger points that refer pain and other symptoms to where the trigger points would usually be found. An example would be trigger points in the gluteal area referring to the lumbar area of the back, when normally lumbar trigger points would refer to the gluteal area. So you may need to check referral areas too, opposite of what the pictures indicate. This is a situation where working with a trained practitioner would be especially helpful.

In the following chapters, the information for each muscle includes lists of common symptoms and factors that may cause or perpetuate trigger points. Again, these are only the most common; you may experience different symptoms, and your causes and perpetuating factors may be different. If you suspect trigger points in a certain muscle but don't see any causes that seem to apply to you, try to imagine whether anything in your life is similar to something on the list, in effect causing the same type of stress on the muscle.

Each muscle chapter provides stretches and, where appropriate, conditioning exercises for the muscle or muscles covered in that chapter. If you're seeing a practitioner, have them check to make sure you're performing the stretches and conditioning exercises properly. Doing them incorrectly could cause additional stress to the muscle. If your symptoms are getting worse, stop doing the self-help techniques and consult with your practitioner.

Conclusion

Once you've determined which two muscles most closely fit your pain pattern, start working on those. Over the next several weeks, add in additional muscles for treatment. Periodically review the guidelines in chapter 8 to make sure you're doing the self-treatments properly. As you start to feel better, you'll develop a clearer picture of which trigger points in which muscles are causing your pain, and which perpetuating factors are reactivating your trigger points.

Head Pain Map

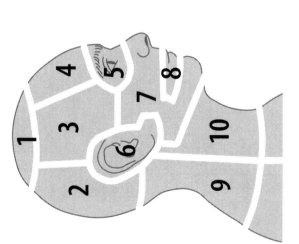

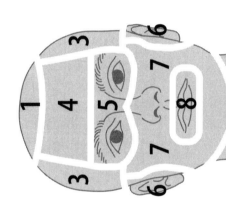

The muscle names are followed by the chapter number

1. Sternocleidomastoid (12)
   Splenius Capitis (11)

2. Trapezius (10)
   Sternocleidomastoid (12)
   Posterior Neck (11)
   Occipitalis (14)
   Digastric (18)
   Temporalis (13)

3. Trapezius (10)
   Sternocleidomastoid (12)
   Temporalis (13)
   Posterior Neck (11)

4. Sternocleidomastoid (12)
   Semispinalis Capitis (11)
   Facial and Scalp (14)

5. Sternocleidomastoid (12)
   Temporalis (13)
   Posterior Neck (11)
   Masseter (15)
   Facial and Scalp (14)
   Trapezius (10)

6. Lateral Pterygoid (16)
   Masseter (15)
   Sternocleidomastoid (12)
   Medial Pterygoid (17)

7. Sternocleidomastoid (12)
   Masseter (15)
   Lateral Pterygoid (16)
   Trapezius (10)
   Digastric (18)
   Medial Pterygoid (17)
   Facial and Scalp (14)

8. Temporalis (13)
   Masseter (14)
   Digastric (18)

9. Trapezius (10)
   Cervical Multifidi (11)
   Splenius Cervicis (11)
   (Also Levator Scapula and Infraspinatus which are not addressed in this book)

10. Sternocleidomastoid (12)
    Digastric (18)
    Medial Pterygoid (17)

Blank Body Chart

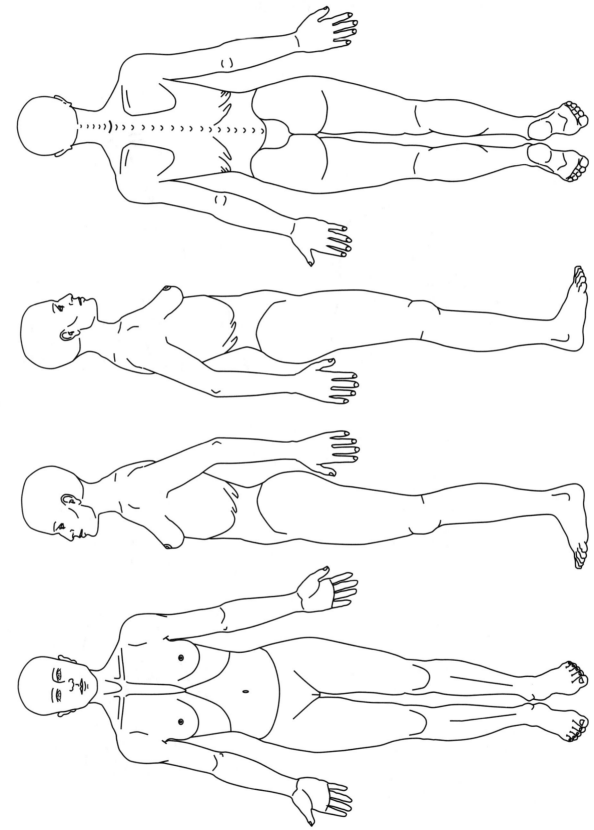

Upper Body Pain Map

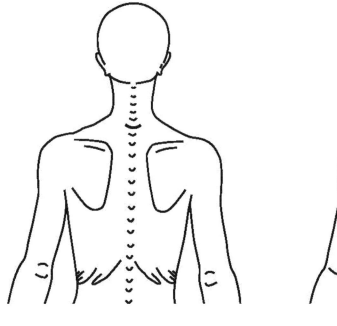

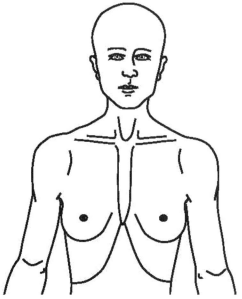

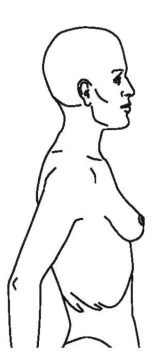

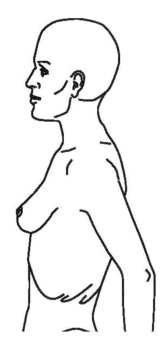

Chapter 10

Trapezius

As you can see from the muscle drawing, the trapezius is a large, kite-shaped muscle covering much of the back and posterior neck. It commonly contains trigger points, and referred pain from these trigger points causes people to seek help more often than for trigger points in any other muscle. Trigger points in the trapezius muscle are a major contributor to headache pain.

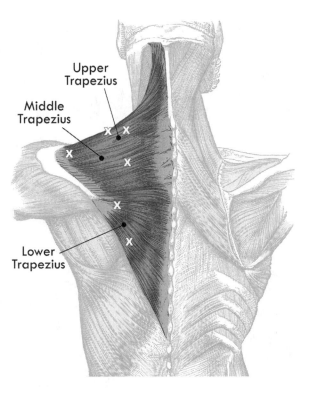

Common Symptoms

There are three main parts to the muscle: the upper, middle, and lower trapezius, and each part has its own actions and common symptoms.

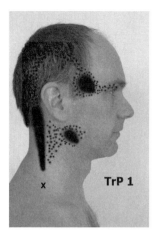

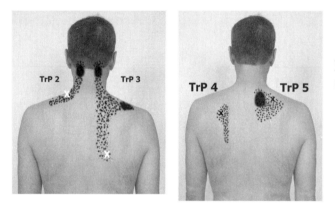

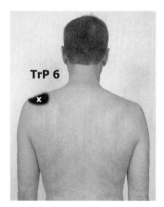

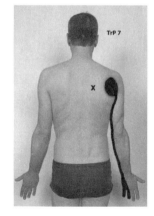

Upper Trapezius
(trigger points #1 and #2)

- Headaches over your temples and/or tension headaches

- Facial, temple, or jaw pain, or pain behind your eye

- Dizziness or vertigo (indicates simultaneous involvement of the sternocleidomastoid muscle, covered in chapter 12)

- Stiffness, limited range of motion, and/or severe pain in your neck

- Intolerance of weight on your shoulders

Middle Trapezius
(trigger points #5 and #6)

- Upper midback pain (trigger point #5 only)

- Superficial burning pain close to your spine (trigger point #5 only)

- Aching pain at the top of your shoulder near the joint (trigger point #6 only)

Lower Trapezius
(trigger points #3, #4, and #7)

- Headaches at the base of your skull (trigger point #3 only)

- Pain in the midback, neck, and/or upper shoulder region

- Possibly referral on the back of your shoulder blade, down the inside of your arm, and into the ring and little fingers—very similar to the referral pattern of the serratus posterior superior, which is not addressed in this book because it does not cause headaches (trigger point #7 only)

- Deep aching and diffuse tenderness over the top of your shoulder (trigger point #3 only)

Possible Causes and Perpetuators

Postural

- Head-forward posture

- Tensing your shoulders

- Cradling a phone between your ear and shoulder

- Sleeping on your front or back with your head rotated to the side for a long period

- Sewing on your lap with your arms unsupported

- Sitting without a firm back support (sitting slumped)

- Bending over for extended periods (for example, if you are a dentist, hygienist, architect, draftsman, or secretary, or have some other job that requires bending over a workspace)

- Carrying a daypack or purse over one shoulder

- Turning your head to one side for long periods to have a conversation or to hear more clearly

Misfitting Furniture or Clothing

- Sitting in a chair without armrests, or with armrests that are too high

- Typing on a keyboard that's too high

- Wearing a bra with straps that are too tight (either the shoulder straps or the torso strap)

- Carrying a purse or daypack that's too heavy

- Wearing a heavy coat

- Walking with a cane that's too long

Medical or Structural

- Getting a whiplash injury (from a car accident, falling on your head, or any sudden jerk of the head)

- Suffering from fatigue

- Having one leg that is shorter than the other

- Having sit bones that aren't level because one side is smaller

- Having short upper arms, which causes you to lean to one side to use armrests

- Having large breasts

- Having tight pectoralis major muscles

Activities

- Sports activities with sudden one-sided movements, such as tennis and golfing

- Jogging

- Playing the violin

- Backpacking

- Bike riding

- Kayaking

Helpful Hints

Putting your hands in your pockets when standing takes the weight off your trapezius muscles. Putting shoulder pads in a heavy coat can help take its weight off the upper trapezius.

If you backpack, try to put most of the weight on your hip strap. If you ride a bike, including a stationary bike, sit as upright as possible by adjusting the handlebars. If you lift weights, avoid excessive amounts of weight and keep your head straight and in alignment with your shoulders, not held forward. If you use a walking cane, be sure it is not so high that it hikes up your shoulder.

Swimming provides good aerobic exercise, but you need to vary your strokes so you don't unduly stress the trapezius muscle. Turning your head to one side, as with the crawl stroke, can aggravate the trapezius.

Self-Help Techniques

Applying Pressure

Trapezius and Paraspinal Pressure

Lie face-up on a firm bed or the floor with your knees bent. Place a tennis ball or racquetball about one inch out to the side of your spine starting at the top of your back, and hold pressure on that spot for eight seconds to one minute. Scoot a small distance to the next spot farther down the back in a line parallel to the spine, and again hold pressure on the spot. Continue working down all the way to the top of the pelvis in order to work on both the trapezius and the paraspinal muscles (the muscles that run in a lengthwise strip on either side of the spine). You may want to repeat this on a second line farther out from the spine, especially if you have a wide back or have tender points farther out. *Do not do this directly on the spine because you may injure yourself!* I recommend using one ball at a time, rather than using a ball on each side at the same time. By performing this technique lying down, as opposed to standing and leaning into a wall, you keep the muscles as passive as possible, since you aren't using them to hold you upright while you're applying pressure.

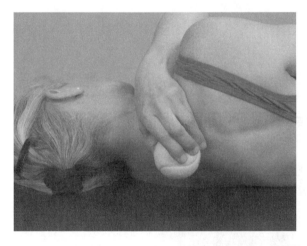

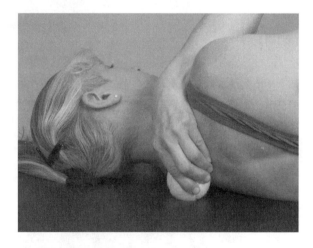

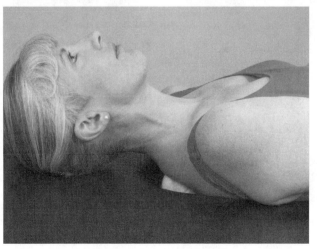

The shading in the following photo marks the area you will want to work on.

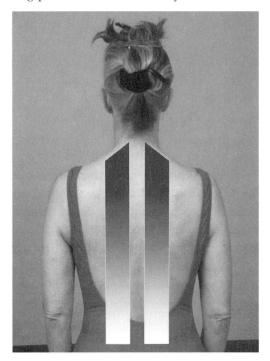

If you are at work or otherwise unable to lie on the floor, I recommend using a Backnobber, available from the Pressure Positive Company (see Resources). Note how both of my hands are pulling the Backnobber away from my body in the direction my fingers are pointing, rather than pressing the Backnobber into the front of my trunk to lever pressure onto my back.

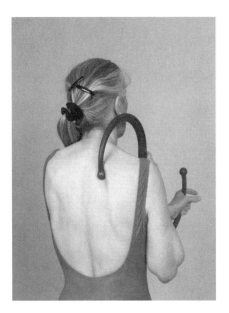

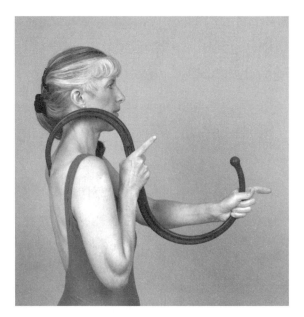

Trapezius Pinch

Place your elbow and forearm on a surface high enough to support the weight of your arm. With the opposite hand, reach across your front and pinch the upper portion of the trapezius muscle. Be sure to stay on the meat of the muscle, and *don't dig your thumb into the depression directly above the collarbone, or you could injure delicate nerves and blood vessels.* You may need to tilt your head slightly toward the side you're working on to keep the muscle relaxed enough to be able to pinch it.

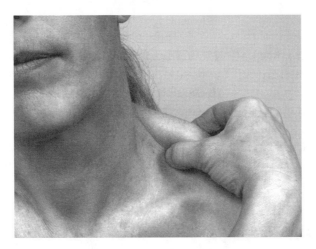

Supraspinatus Pressure

Pressure on the supraspinatus muscle will help treat the upper trapezius. Stand in a doorway and place a tennis ball in the groove of the doorjamb at about hip level, holding onto the ball with the hand of the side opposite the one you're working. Bend over at about 90 degrees, and be sure to let your head go completely limp. With the ball pressing against the top of your shoulder, lean into the ball with however much pressure you want to apply. While still holding onto the ball with your opposite hand and continuing to keep your head fully relaxed, work spots across the top of your shoulder.

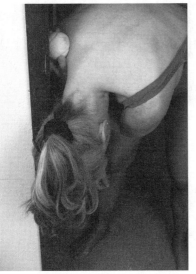 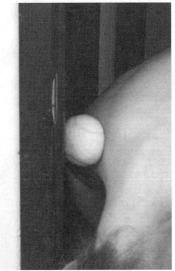

Posterior Neck Pressure

See chapter 11, Posterior Neck Muscles, for details on this self-treatment. Perform the treatment on the back of your neck using a golf ball.

Stretches

Trapezius Stretch

This stretch benefits the middle and lower trapezius. Lie on your back with your arms at your sides, then move your arms through the positions indicated in the photographs: Raise your arms so your upper arms are perpendicular to the floor and your forearms are parallel to the floor, with your elbows bent at a 90-degree angle. Then, while still holding a 90-degree angle at your elbows, lower your hands so they touch the surface above your head. Next, extend your arms out straight above your head, palms up. Next, slide your upper arms down until they're perpendicular to your trunk and your elbows are again bent at approximately a 90-degree angle, so your forearms are parallel to your trunk. Last, bring your arms down to your sides and take two deep breaths. Repeat three to five times.

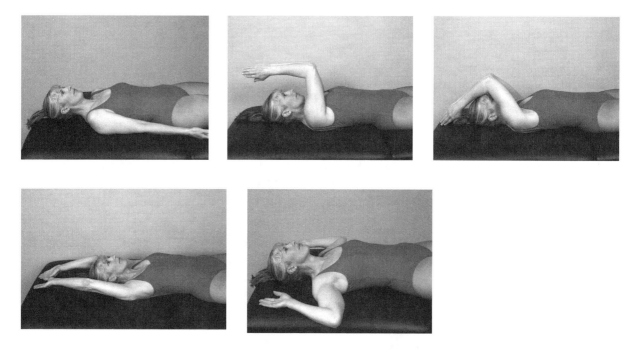

Posterior Neck Stretch

See chapter 11, Posterior Neck Muscles, for details on how to do this stretch.

Pectoralis Stretch

Stretching the pectoralis will benefit the trapezius. Stand in a doorway with your arm outstretched at a 90-degree angle from your body. Raise your forearm and place it along the door frame, including your elbow. With the foot of the same side placed about one step forward, rotate your body gently away from the side you're stretching.

Move your forearm up so that your upper arm is at about a 45-degree angle to the door frame and stretch.

Bring your forearm down below the first position and stretch. Each position will stretch a different part of the muscle.

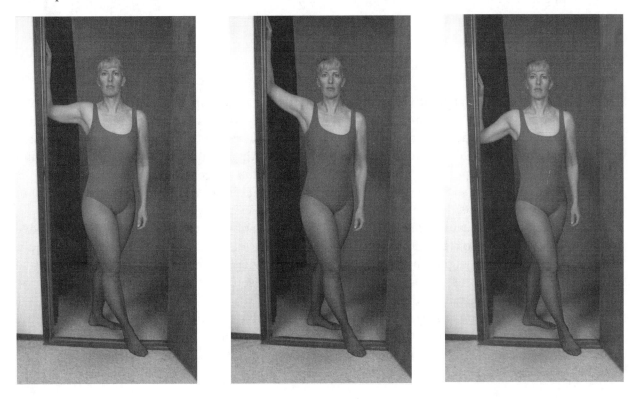

Exercises

Jump rope. Jump rope while moving forward.

Proper posture. To learn proper posture and reduce head-forward posture, see "Head-Forward Posture" in chapter 5, Body Mechanics.

Also See

- Chapter 12, Sternocleidomastoid

- Chapter 13, Temporalis (satellite trigger points)

- Chapter 14, Facial and Scalp Muscles (occipitalis, satellite trigger points)

- Chapter 11, Posterior Neck Muscles (satellite trigger points)

- Chapter 15, Masseter (satellite trigger points)

Conclusion

Trigger points in the supraspinatus may keep trapezius trigger points active. Trigger points in the levator scapulae, infraspinatus, and rhomboid muscles may keep trapezius trigger points active and may also have referral patterns similar to those of the trapezius muscle. Trigger points in the pectoralis major and pectoralis minor muscles may cause those muscles to tighten up and put a strain on the mid and upper back, therefore keeping trapezius trigger points active. Trigger points in the serratus posterior superior have a referral pattern that is similar to trapezius trigger point #7. It is worthwhile to consider that these muscles may have trigger points that need to be relieved. Since they don't directly cause headaches or TMJ pain, none of the trigger points mentioned above are addressed in this book, but if you can't relieve your headaches with the self-help techniques in this book after six to eight weeks, you may wish to consider treating trigger points in these muscles. See the Resources section for books and other resources that can provide guidance on self-treatment of muscles not covered in this book.

If you suspected trapezius trigger points but were unable to relieve your symptoms with the self-help techniques in this chapter, you may need to see a doctor to rule out occipital neuralgia or cervicogenic headaches. You may need to see a chiropractor or osteopathic physician to determine whether you have vertebrae out of alignment.

Chapter 11

Posterior Neck Muscles

It is likely that the muscles in the back of your neck will be some of the most important for you to treat in order to resolve headaches. Quite a few muscles are located in the back of your neck: the splenius capitis, splenius cervicis, cervical multifidi, semispinalis cervicis, semispinalis capitis, and the suboccipitals.

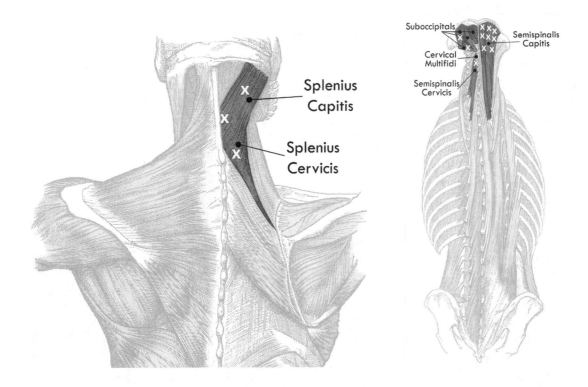

Common Symptoms

The photographs demonstrate the common referral patterns, but note that headaches can be a composite of trigger point pain referral patterns from various muscles of the neck and in and around the mouth and jaw, so you may need to treat several muscles to relieve your pain.

Splenius Capitis

- Pain on the top of your head, but slightly toward the side of the trigger point

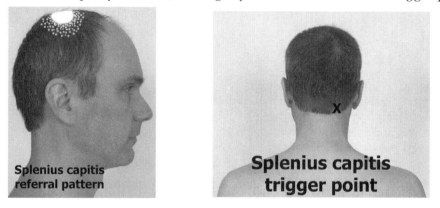

Splenius capitis referral pattern

Splenius capitis trigger point

Splenius Cervicis

- Diffuse pain throughout the inside of your head

- Pain focused behind your eye or shooting through your head to the back of your eye

- Pain at the back of your skull

- Pain at the junction of your neck and the top of your shoulder and up the back of your neck

- Blurring of near vision on the same side as the trigger point

- Neck stiffness

- Limited range of motion

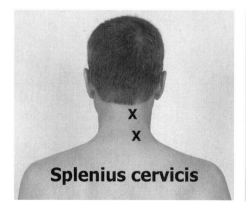

Splenius cervicis

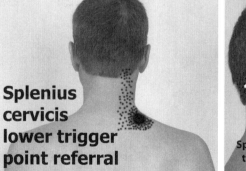

Splenius cervicis lower trigger point referral

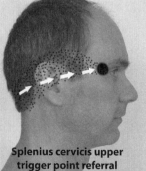

Splenius cervicis upper trigger point referral

Cervical Multifidi, Semispinalis Cervicis, and Semispinalis Capitis

- You feel pain and tenderness over the back of your head and neck.

- The pressure of lying on a pillow is very painful.

- Range of motion is painful and restricted in all directions, with the pain worse when you bend your head forward.

- If the greater occipital nerve becomes entrapped, symptoms may also include numbness, tingling, and burning pain on the back of your head.

- Please note that the semispinalis cervicis trigger point is in the same location as the middle semispinalis capitis trigger point, but the semispinalis capitis is more superficial, while the semispinalis cervicis is deeper.

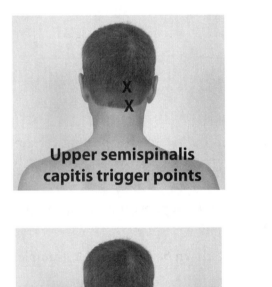

Upper semispinalis capitis trigger points

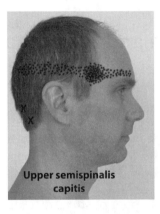

Upper semispinalis capitis

Multifidi

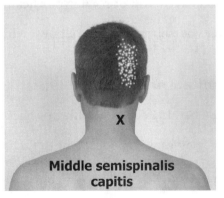

Middle semispinalis capitis

Suboccipitals

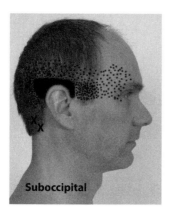

Suboccipital

- You feel referred pain inside your head, but it is difficult for you to define a specific area.

- The pain is vaguely more localized from the back of your skull, over your ear, and to your temples, forehead, and eye.

- The pressure of lying on a pillow is very painful.

- You feel soreness just below the base of your skull.

Possible Causes and Perpetuators

Postural

- Head-forward posture

- Holding your neck in an awkward position, as when bird-watching, playing certain musical instruments, looking up for a long period of time, or falling asleep on the couch with your head propped up on the arm

- Sitting at a desk with poor posture, including lack of lumbar support and placing papers where you have to tilt or rotate your head to look at them

- Propping yourself up on your elbows while lying face-down on the floor, for example, to watch TV

Misfitting Furniture or Clothing

- Wearing a bathing cap, coat, shirt, or necktie that is too tight

- Using eyeglasses with a focal length that's too short

Medical or Structural

- Holding your neck forward as compensation for an excessive outward spinal curve in your midback (kyphosis), which can be aggravated by tension in the pectoralis major muscles

- Getting a whiplash injury, which may be especially detrimental if your head was rotated at the time of the accident

- Falling on your head

- Having vertebrae that are out of alignment, causing nerve entrapment

- Having a long neck

- Getting a laminectomy (a type of spine surgery)

- Having cervical facet joint osteoarthritis, which particularly affects the semispinalis capitis

Activities

- Diving into a pool

- Pulling on a rope or lifting heavy weights, particularly with your head rotated or held forward

Other

- Exposure to a cold draft, such as from air-conditioning, when the muscle is fatigued

- Depression

Helpful Hints

Read through chapter 5, Body Mechanics, paying particular attention to the sections "Mechanical Stressors" and "Head-Forward Posture." Following the self-help suggestions in those sections will greatly help with trigger points in your neck. Don't do exercises that involve rolling your head.

Avoid cold drafts, and keep your neck warm by wearing a scarf, turtleneck, or neck gaiter. You may even need to wear something around your neck while sleeping.

If you're depressed, you may be rounding your shoulders and holding your head forward. Treat the underlying cause of depression with counseling, acupuncture, homeopathic remedies, and/or herbs. See the section "Emotional Factors" in chapter 7, Other Perpetuating Factors, for more details.

Self-Help Techniques

Applying Pressure

I find it most effective to treat the trapezius muscles first, and then the posterior neck muscles. Read through chapter 10, Trapezius, and at a minimum do the trapezius and paraspinal pressure technique prior to working on the muscles in the back of your neck.

Posterior Neck Pressure

To treat the back of your neck, use a golf ball and lie face-up with your hands behind your neck. One palm should be squarely over the other palm, with the golf ball in the center of your top

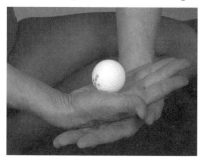

palm, *not* where the fingers join the palm. Keep your head relaxed throughout the self-treatment.

To apply pressure, rotate your head toward the ball. Be sure to work on the muscles to the side of the spine; *don't put the ball directly on the spine because you may injure yourself!* To move the ball, roll your head away from the side you're working on, move the ball a small distance, then rotate your head back toward the side you're working on. If you want more pressure, rotate your head even farther; if you want less pressure, don't rotate your head as far. *Don't pick your head up to move the ball.* This will place additional stress on the muscles. Be sure to move the ball by rotating your head away from the ball.

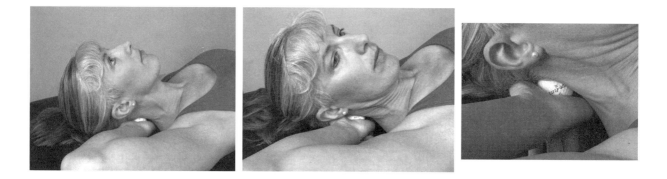

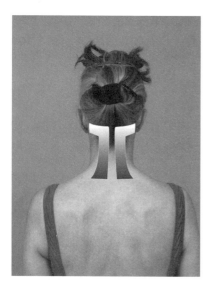

The shading in the image to the left marks the area you will want to work on. You may work along the base of the skull and down the back of the neck. Try to get all the way to the base of the neck, where it intersects the top of the shoulder; this will work on the entire splenius cervicis muscle.

Stretches

Posterior Neck Stretch

You may do this stretch under a hot shower and, if possible, seated on a stool. Lock your fingers behind your head and pull your head gently forward. Bring your head back up. Turn your head to one side at a 45-degree angle and gently pull your head in that direction. Bring your head back up again. Place one hand on the top of your head and gently pull your head down to that side. Repeat the entire sequence on the opposite side.

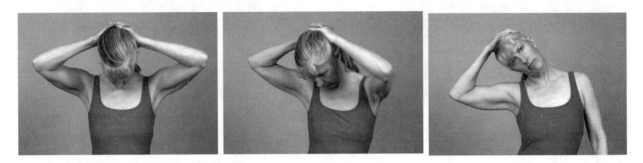

Side-Bending Neck Stretch

Lie face-up. Tuck your left hand under your buttocks, palm down, and place your right hand on top of your head. Looking straight up at the ceiling, gently pull your head down toward your right shoulder.

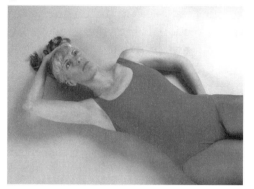 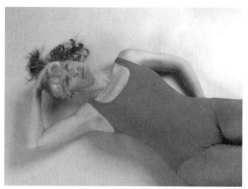

Next, rotate your head 45 degrees to the right and gently pull your head down toward your right shoulder.

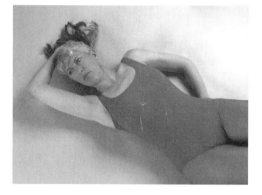 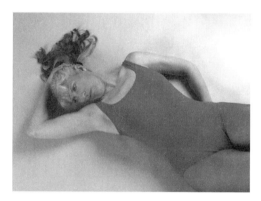

And finally, rotate your head 45 degrees to the left, and again gently pull your head down toward your *right* shoulder. Switch hands and repeat the same stretches on the opposite side, gently pulling your head down toward your left shoulder.

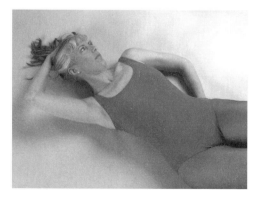 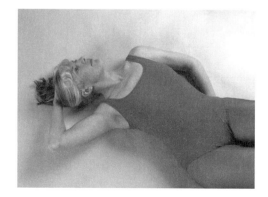

Also See

- Chapter 18, Digastric (posterior portion)

- Chapter 12, Sternocleidomastoid

- Chapter 10, Trapezius

Conclusion

Trigger points in the levator scapulae, infraspinatus, and some of the paraspinal muscles may keep posterior neck muscle trigger points active, and they also have referral patterns similar to those of the muscles in the back of the neck. Trigger points in the pectoralis major muscles may cause it to tighten up and put a strain on the mid and upper back, therefore keeping trapezius trigger points active, and then affecting the neck. It is worthwhile to consider that there may be trigger points in these muscles that need to be relieved. Since they don't directly cause headaches or TMJ pain, none of the trigger points mentioned above are addressed in this book, but if you can't relieve your headaches with the self-help techniques in this book after six to eight weeks, you may wish to consider treating trigger points in these muscles. See the Resources section for books and other resources that can provide guidance on self-treatment of the muscles not covered in this book.

If you suspected trigger points in your posterior neck muscles but were unable to relieve your symptoms with the self-help techniques in this chapter, you may need to see a doctor to rule out several types of arthritis, herniated or bulging disks, or stenosis. Or you may have vertebrae out of alignment; a chiropractor or osteopathic physician can evaluate and treat this condition.

Chapter 12

Sternocleidomastoid

The sternocleidomastoid muscle has two heads, the sternal and clavicular divisions. Each head has different referral patterns, and some of their typical symptoms are different as well. Trigger points in the sternocleidomastoid are a frequent cause of headaches.

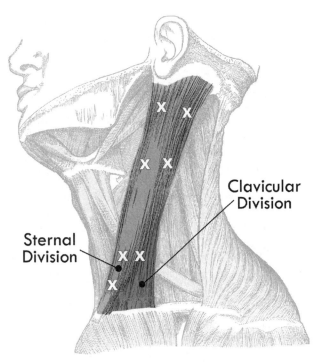

Common Symptoms

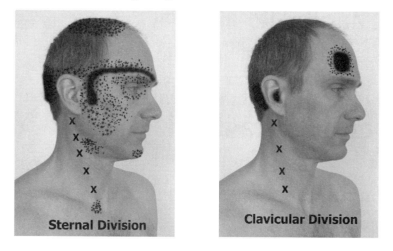

Sternal Division

Clavicular Division

Both the Sternal and Clavicular Divisions

- You have tension headaches.

- You have a persistent dry, tickling cough.

- The muscles may be sore to the touch.

- Entrapment of certain cranial nerves by the sternocleidomastoid may cause partial paralysis of the trapezius on the same side.

Sternal Division Only

- Referred pain to the top of your head, the back of your head, your cheek, or over the top of or behind your eye

- Sinus congestion on the affected side

- Referred symptoms to your eye and sinuses

- Pain in your cheek and molars on the affected side

- A chronic sore throat (due to referred pain to your throat and the back of your tongue when swallowing, rather than infection)

- Profuse tearing of your eye

- Reddening of the whites of your eyes and the insides of your eyelids

- Visual disturbances, including blurred vision or dimming of perceived light intensity

- A drooping upper eyelid

- Eyelid twitching

- One-sided deafness, a partial loss of hearing, or a crackling sound in your ear

Clavicular Division Only

- Headaches on your forehead, possibly across your whole forehead rather than just on one side

- Earaches (deep pain)

- Dizziness and disturbed balance (disorientation) or vertigo (a spinning sensation), especially when changing position

- Nausea and loss of appetite

- Propensity to seasickness or car sickness

- Veering into doorjambs or objects on the affected side

- Veering to the side when driving

- Inability to gauge differences in weights held in your hands

- Sweating, blanching, and a cool sensation on your forehead

Possible Causes and Perpetuators

Postural

- Head-forward posture

- Constantly tilting your head to avoid light reflections on your glasses or contacts, or to improve hearing

- Looking up for long periods of time, such as in overhead work like painting a ceiling

- Tilting your head back or turning it to the side for long periods

- Reading in bed with a light off to the side, as you will likely keep your head turned to the side to see better

Misfitting Furniture or Clothing

- Using a pillow that's too high

- Wearing a necktie or a collar that's too tight (a finger should fit comfortably inside your shirt collar, even when your head is turned)

Medical or Structural

- Having a chronic cough

- Breathing improperly

- Getting a whiplash injury (from a car accident, falling on your head, or any sudden jerk of your head)

- Having a chronic infection, such as sinusitis, a dental abscess, or oral herpes (cold sores)

- Getting an acute infection, such as the common cold or flu, which can activate latent trigger points

- Having a tight pectoralis major muscle pulling down and forward on your collarbone

- Having a severe deformity or injury that restricts upper body movement, forcing your neck to overcompensate to keep balance

- Having one leg shorter than the other

- Having sit bones that aren't level because one side is smaller

- Having severe scoliosis (a curved and/or rotated spine)

- Leakage of cerebrospinal fluid following a spinal tap, which can activate sternocleido-mastoid trigger points and subsequently cause a chronic headache that may last from weeks to years

Activities

- Horseback riding and horse handling

- Swimming (turning your head to breathe)

- Drinking alcohol (hangover headaches as a result of alcohol stimulating trigger points in your sternocleidomastoid)

Helpful Hints

Postural

Read through chapter 5, Body Mechanics, paying particular attention to the sections "Mechanical Stressors" and "Head-Forward Posture." Following the self-help suggestions in those sections will greatly help with trigger points in your neck.

When lying down, don't lead with your head when you get up. First roll onto your side or front, then use your arms to get you started. When turning over in bed at night, roll your head on the pillow instead of lifting it. When sleeping, try to keep your head facing in the same direction as your torso, rather than turned to the side. Don't use an older-style large-celled foam pillow, as this type of foam causes jiggling and vibration. However, the newer memory foam pillows, which have denser cells, are a good option. Your pillow should support your head at a level that keeps your spine in alignment and is comfortable when you lie on your side.

Reading in bed isn't a good idea, but if you aren't willing to give this up, at least make sure your light is located directly overhead, on either the headboard or the ceiling. Again, keep your head facing in the same direction as your torso, rather than turned to the side. A comfortable chair next to the bed, with appropriate lighting, is even better.

Avoid headrests that push your head forward. A lumbar support may help restore normal lumbar and cervical curves. Get a headset or speaker for your phone. If you type, the copy should be as close as possible to the side of the computer screen so that you don't have to rotate your head to the side for long periods of time. Orthotic inserts in your shoes may improve your standing posture. Take whatever steps are necessary to correct your vision or reduce visual stress, as you may be holding your head forward to read and see.

Medical or Structural

If you have a physical asymmetry, such as a small hemipelvis (sit bones), a short leg, or short upper arms, see a specialist to get compensating lifts or pads. Chiropractic adjustments, acupuncture, and massage can help reduce scoliosis.

Chronic infections must be eliminated or controlled as much as possible. You will probably need to work on your sternocleidomastoid muscles after illnesses such as a cold, the flu, or cold sores (a herpes outbreak). A chronic cough from asthma or emphysema can aggravate trigger points, as can breathing improperly.

Activities

If you swim, avoid the crawl stroke, or any stroke that requires you to turn your head to one side to breathe. *Don't do head-rolling exercises!* In particular, don't bend or roll your head backward. Also, avoid any overhead work that requires you to bend your head backward. If you're doing the pectoralis stretch from chapter 10, Trapezius, be sure to keep your head back over your shoulders throughout the exercise and look straight forward (with your nose in a line with your breast bone).

Self-Help Techniques

Applying Pressure

Sternocleidomastoid Pressure

It is best to do this self-treatment lying down, but you can do it sitting up, which comes in handy at work. Tilt your head just a little toward the side you're working on, bringing your ear closer to your shoulder, then rotate your head slightly *away* from that side. If you place your fingers in the spots indicated in the photos, you will know when your head is positioned correctly, because your fingers will be closer to each other instead of further apart.

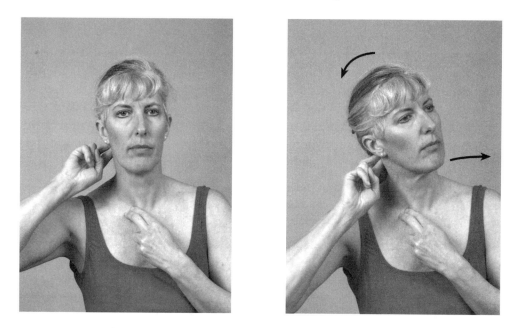

To work the lower half of the muscle, grasp *both parts* of the muscle with the hand on the same side (for example, use your right hand to grasp the right sternocleidomastoid), but *don't dig your fingers deep into your neck or you could injure delicate nerves and blood vessels!* Pinch and pull at the same time, holding each tender spot eight seconds to one minute.

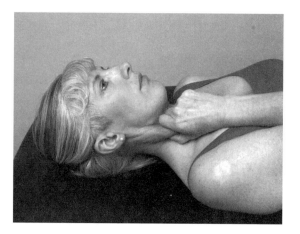

To work the upper half of the muscle, switch hands (for example, use your left hand to grasp the upper half of your right sternocleidomastoid) and pull the muscle outward in the middle. Then use the hand on the same side to work your way up to the attachment behind the ear. For most people, this is the tightest part but also the most critical to work on. If your sternocleidomastoid is particularly tight, it may be hard to get ahold of it at first. But after you've worked on it a few times, it should become easier to grasp. Remember that you may have to work this muscle again after you're sick, because its trigger points will likely be reactivated by certain illnesses.

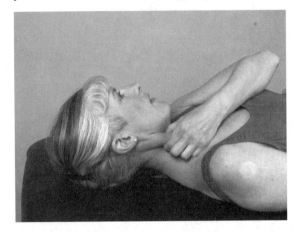 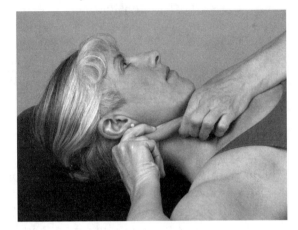

Stretches

Side-Bending Neck Stretch

You'll find complete instructions for this stretch in chapter 11, Posterior Neck Muscles.

Proper Breathing

Place one hand on your chest and the other on your belly. When you inhale, both hands should rise. As you exhale, both hands should fall. You need to train yourself to notice when you're breathing only into your chest and make sure you start breathing into your belly.

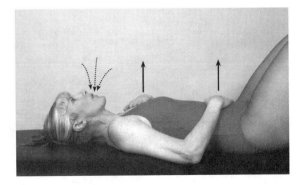 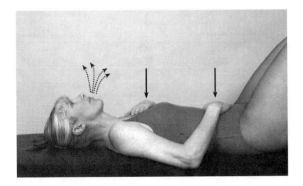

Also See

- Chapter 10, Trapezius

- Chapter 15, Masseter (satellite trigger points)

- Chapter 14, Facial and Scalp Muscles (platysma, and satellite trigger points caused by the sternocleidomastoid)

- Chapter 11, Posterior Neck Muscles

- Chapter 13, Temporalis (satellite trigger points)

Conclusion

Trigger points in the levator scapulae, pectoralis major, scalene, and sternalis muscles may keep sternocleidomastoid muscle trigger points active, so it is worthwhile to consider that there may be trigger points in these muscles that need to be relieved. Since they don't directly cause headaches or TMJ pain, these trigger points are not addressed in this book, but if you can't relieve your headaches with the self-help techniques in this book after six to eight weeks, you may wish to consider treating trigger points in these muscles. See the Resources section for books and other resources that can provide guidance on self-treatment of muscles not covered in this book.

If you suspected trigger points in your sternocleidomastoid but were unable to relieve your symptoms with the self-help techniques in this chapter, you may need to see a doctor to rule out causes other than trigger points, including atypical facial neuralgia, trigeminal neuralgia, dizziness caused by problems within the ears, Ménière's disease, arthritis of the sternoclavicular joint, and wryneck (where the neck is twisted to the side due to muscle spasms).

Chapter 13

Temporalis

Trigger points in the temporalis are fairly common. Tenderness in your temporalis may indicate trigger points, but even in the absence of tenderness, trigger points may be present and causing symptoms. Try putting the knuckles of the index and middle finger of your nondominant hand in your mouth vertically—if you can't get both in, you have trigger points in your temporalis and/or masseter muscles.

If your jaw makes grating or popping sounds, you may have disk erosion, bone on bone due to complete loss of the disk, or arthritis. This can be caused by long-term trigger points that have not been relieved, so it is important to inactivate trigger points before permanent damage results. You may need to see a specialist in temporomandibular joint evaluation. Be sure to inactivate trigger points in your mouth and temporalis muscle areas prior to dental intervention because your bite may change from trigger point work. (For full details, see "Self-Help for TMJ Dysfunction" in chapter 4.)

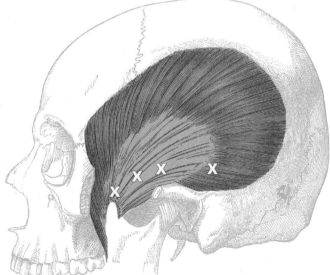

Common Symptoms

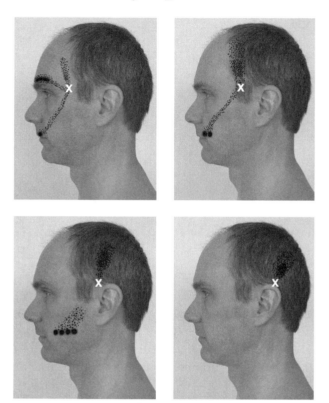

- You may have referred pain on and above your temple and ear, over your eyebrow, to your upper teeth on the affected side, and occasionally to your face and jaw joint, usually experienced as a headache or toothache.

- Your teeth can become sensitive to heat or cold, or achy.

- You may have improper bite alignment.

- Though clenching your teeth is often a cause of temporalis trigger points, it may also be caused by trigger points.

- Your jaw may zigzag during opening and closing.

Possible Causes and Perpetuators

Postural

- Head-forward posture

Misfitting Furniture or Clothing

- Wearing a surgical mask, respirator, or anything that fits tightly on your face

Medical or Structural

- Keeping your mouth open for long periods, such as during dental work

- Receiving a direct blow to the side of your head

- Cervical traction without a bite splint

- Chronic infections or inflammation, even after the infection or inflammation has been resolved

- Systemic perpetuating factors, such as a folate deficiency, hypothyroidism, or serum levels of thyroid hormones (T3 and T4) in the low-normal range

Other

- Clenching your jaw or grinding your teeth

- Chewing gum

- Teeth making contact prematurely and throwing off your bite (this may start after dental work)

- A cold draft on the side of your head, such as from a car window or air-conditioning

- Satellite trigger points caused by trigger points in your trapezius and/or sternocleido-mastoid muscles

Helpful Hints

To learn proper posture, see "Head-Forward Posture" in chapter 5, Body Mechanics. Be sure to evaluate and eliminate any systemic perpetuating factors, such as nutritional deficiencies and reduced thyroid function (discussed in chapters 6 and 7). Folic acid, calcium, or magnesium deficiency may be a cause of teeth grinding.

A displaced jaw disk may cause a feeling of pressure, leading you to bite down in an attempt to relieve the pressure, but this only adds to the problem. You will need to see a dental specialist for evaluation. Avoid chewing gum, or other chewy or hard foods. If you wear a close-fitting face mask of any kind, remove it periodically and stretch your jaw.

Any body asymmetries need to be corrected, whether by heel lifts, good-quality orthotic foot-beds, massage, or chiropractic treatments, since these problems activate posterior neck trigger points, which then cause satellite trigger points in muscles in and around your mouth. Mouth breathing, too, needs to be eliminated by correcting the causes, such as a nasal obstruction.

Protect your head from drafts by wearing a scarf or hat that covers the sides of your head. Applying a hot pack to your temple area and the side of your face may offer some relief. Trigger points in the trapezius, posterior neck, and sternocleidomastoid muscles can keep temporalis trigger points active, so you'll need to treat any trigger points in those areas to obtain lasting relief.

Self-Help Techniques

Applying Pressure

Temporalis Pressure

Using your fingertips, apply pressure to the areas above your temple and ear. While holding the tender points, slowly open and close your jaw. Move to another tender point and slowly open and close your jaw. Repeat for any tender points on the sides of your head.

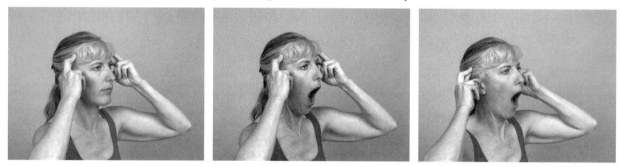

Look at the anatomical drawing and the referral pattern photos to make sure you're working on the whole muscle. It covers most of the side of your head.

Stretches

Yawning

Yawn widely to stretch the temporalis muscle.

Temporalis Stretch

After applying hot packs to the sides of your head, lie face-up. Insert your index finger behind your lower front teeth and pull forward and down, giving the muscles crossing your jaw joint a gentle stretch. This is a good stretch to do just before bedtime.

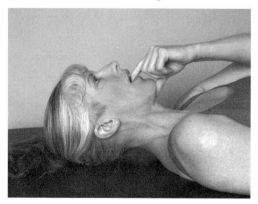 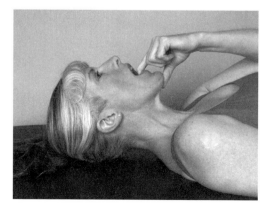

If your jaw deviates to one side, add the following stretch. If it deviates to the left, place your right fingers on your right cheek over your upper teeth and your left fingers on your lower jaw on your left side. Push your lower jaw toward the right. If your jaw deviates toward the right, do the opposite motion.

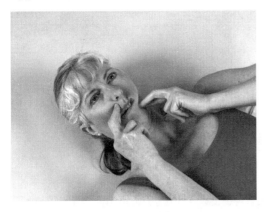
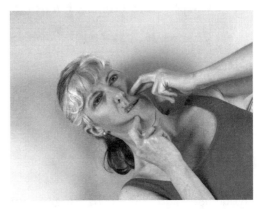

Exercises

Temporalis Exercise

Once your temporalis trigger points have been inactivated for a few weeks, for conditioning and strengthening you may perform the above stretches with *gentle* resistance by pressing your jaw very slightly against your fingers at the same time you are pushing your jaw to the opposite side.

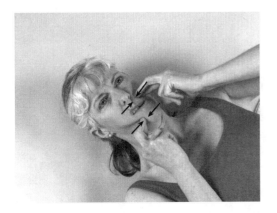
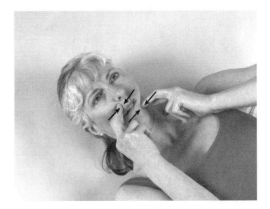

Tongue Rolls

Tongue rolls help relax the muscles of the mouth. For complete instructions for this exercise, see the section "Abuse of Muscles" in chapter 5, Body Mechanics.

Also See

- Chapter 10, Trapezius (upper portion of the muscle)

- Chapter 12, Sternocleidomastoid

- Chapter 15, Masseter

- Chapter 17, Medial Pterygoid

- Chapter 16, Lateral Pterygoid

Conclusion

If you suspected temporalis trigger points but were unable to relieve your symptoms with the self-help techniques in this chapter, you may need to see a dentist or other specialist in TMJ disorders. A bite guard or occlusal splint with a flat occlusal plane may help, but again, try to inactivate any trigger points in this area first, as doing so can change your bite. You may also need to see a dentist or doctor to rule out temporomandibular joint internal displacements, diseased teeth, polymyalgia rheumatica, temporal arteritis, or temporal tendinitis.

Chapter 14

Facial and Scalp Muscles

Several muscles in your face and scalp can cause or contribute to headache and TMJ pain: the orbicularis oculi, zygomaticus major, platysma, buccinator, frontalis, and occipitalis. Primary trigger points can form in these muscles due to habitual facial expressions, any of the factors that lead to TMJ pain, or any systemic perpetuating factors. Or satellite trigger points can form via symptoms referred by the trapezius and neck muscles.

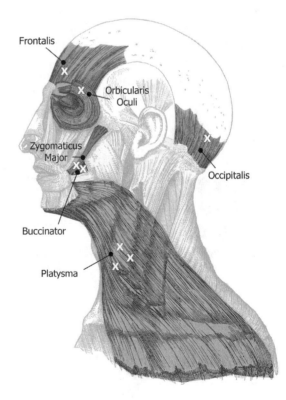

Common Symptoms

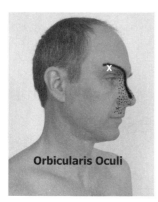

Orbicularis Oculi

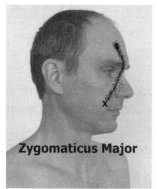

Zygomaticus Major

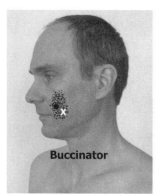

Buccinator

Orbicularis Oculi

- Referral from the orbicularis oculi travels over your eyebrow and down your nose, possibly spilling off your nose and into your upper lip.

- You may be unable to close your eye tightly, causing your eye to be dry.

- Tears may not drain properly and may spill over your lower eyelid.

- When reading type with strong black and white contrast, such as a book, the letters may seem to jump.

- You may have difficulty looking up without tilting your head backward, since your eyelid won't go up all the way.

Zygomaticus Major

- The zygomaticus major refers pain from below your cheek, up next to your nose, and into your forehead.

- You may have difficulty smiling or laughing.

- You may have a restriction of your jaw opening by 10 to 20 millimeters less than normal.

Buccinator

- Referral from the buccinator feels both superficial and deep under your cheekbone and is worse with chewing.

- You may have difficulty whistling or playing a wind instrument.

- You may perceive that you have difficulty swallowing, even though your ability to swallow is actually normal.

Frontalis

- You may feel pain over your forehead in the area of the trigger point.

- Trigger points in the middle half of the frontalis can entrap the supraorbital nerve, causing a headache in your forehead.

Occipitalis

- Referred pain may cause one-sided headaches.

- You may have pain between the top of your ear and the top of your head.

- You may have pain deep in your head, and intense pain deep behind your eye, in your eye, and in your eyelid.

- You may have pain when lying on a pillow because of pressure against the muscles.

Platysma

- The platysma refers a strange pain like multiple pinpricks over your cheek and the lower part of your face. One of its trigger points, located close to the collarbone, may refer hot prickling pain across the front of your chest.

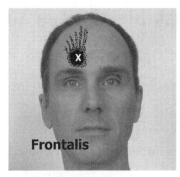

Frontalis

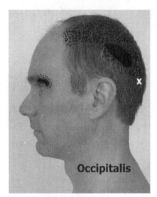

Occipitalis

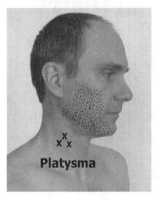

Platysma

Possible Causes and Perpetuators

- Habitual frowning or squinting may cause trigger points in the orbicularis oculi.

- Trigger points from the sternal division of the sternocleidomastoid may cause satellite trigger points in the orbicularis oculi.

- Trigger points in the chewing muscles that are severe enough to restrict your ability to open your mouth may activate trigger points in the zygomaticus major.

- Trigger points in the buccinator may be activated by dental appliances that don't fit well, such as a bite guard that needs to be replaced.

- Frontalis trigger points are likely to be satellite trigger points that develop because of referral from the clavicular division of the sternocleidomastoid. They may also result from raising your eyebrows frequently and wrinkling your forehead.

- Occipitalis trigger points form as a result of squinting due to either deterioration of vision or glaucoma. They may also be satellite trigger points from referred pain from your posterior neck muscles.

Helpful Hints

Pain from trigger points in the orbicularis oculi, zygomaticus, and buccinator is frequently diagnosed as a tension headache. It may also be misdiagnosed as temporomandibular joint dysfunction, which needs to be ruled out.

Pain from trigger points in the frontalis and occipitalis is also frequently diagnosed as a tension headache. Be sure to also check the sternocleidomastoid, digastric (posterior portion), and semispinalis cervicis (one of the posterior neck muscles), since trigger points in these muscles can activate trigger points in your forehead or the back of your head.

Trigger points in the platysma are rarely present without trigger points in the sternocleidomastoid or scalene muscles, or the muscles used for chewing (the masseter, digastric, medial pterygoid, lateral pterygoid, and temporalis muscles), so be sure to check those muscles for trigger points also.

Avoid holding facial expressions for long periods of time, such as wrinkling your forehead, raising your eyebrows, or frowning. You probably aren't aware that you are doing this, so you need to train yourself to notice it, then relax. Scalp and face massages can help relax the muscles and increase circulation.

Self-Help Techniques

Applying Pressure

Orbicularis Oculi Pressure

To treat the orbicularis oculi, use the tip of your index finger to press in the area below the eyebrow, on the bone above your eye. You may also pinch and roll the muscle between your thumb and index finger; just pinch as close to the bone as possible to be sure you're getting ahold of the muscle in addition to the skin.

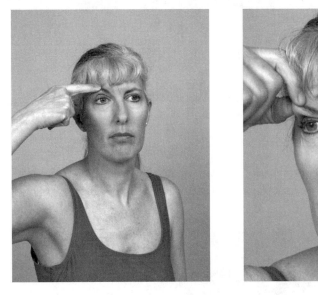

Buccinator and Zygomaticus Major Pressure

To treat the buccinator and the zygomaticus major, put the thumb of your opposite hand inside your mouth and the index finger outside your mouth. Pinch from just below the lower rim of your cheekbone down to close to the bottom of your jaw. You may stretch your cheek outward as you do this, and open your mouth wider as the trigger points release.

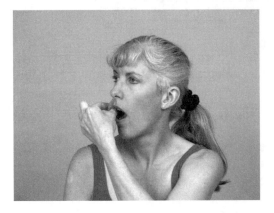
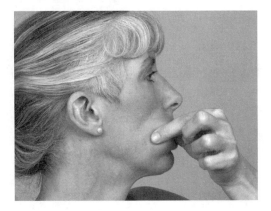

Frontalis Pressure

Use your fingers to press on frontalis trigger points on your forehead.

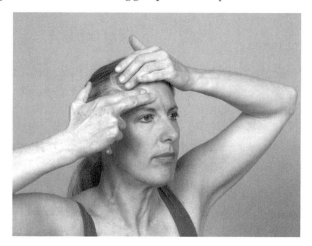

Occipitalis Pressure

Use your fingers to search for trigger points on the back of your head in the occipitalis muscle. You may also rest your head on a tennis ball. Lie on your back, place the tennis ball between your head and the floor or bed, and rest your head on it.

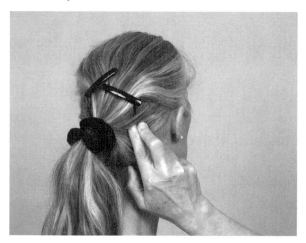

Platysma

The muscles and other structures in the front of the neck are very delicate, so it's probably best to have a trained therapist treat the platysma. Trigger points in the platysma are uncommon.

Exercises

Tongue Rolls

Tongue rolls help relax the muscles of the mouth. For complete instructions for this exercise, see the section "Abuse of Muscles" in chapter 5, Body Mechanics.

Also See

- Chapter 12, Sternocleidomastoid

- Chapter 15, Masseter

- Chapter 16, Lateral Pterygoid

- Chapter 17, Medial Pterygoid

- Chapter 18, Digastric

- Chapter 10, Trapezius

- Chapter 13, Temporalis

- Chapter 11, Posterior Neck Muscles (semispinalis cervicis)

Conclusion

Trigger points in the scalene muscles may keep trigger points in the facial muscles active, so it is worthwhile to consider that there may be scalene trigger points that need to be relieved. Since they don't directly cause headaches or TMJ pain, the trigger points mentioned above are not addressed in this book, but if you can't relieve your headaches with the self-help techniques in this book after six to eight weeks, you may wish to consider treating trigger points in the scalene muscles. See the Resources section for books and other resources that can provide guidance on self-treatment of muscles not covered in this book.

Chapter 15

Masseter

Trigger points are very common in the masseter, a powerful muscle used primarily for chewing. Chewing gum or grinding your teeth increases the likelihood of trigger points. Dental work can change your bite, and this, too, can cause trigger points. Long procedures, including the removal of wisdom teeth, are especially problematic, as they require overstretching, which can cause trauma to the muscles and initiate trigger points.

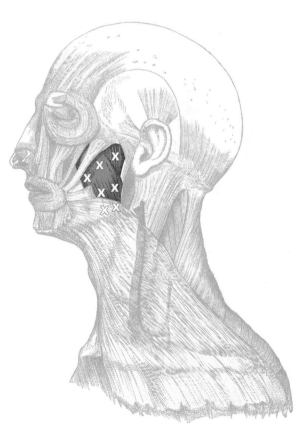

Common Symptoms

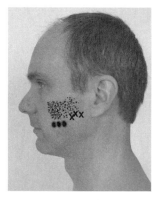

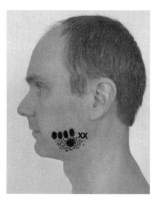

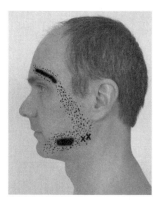

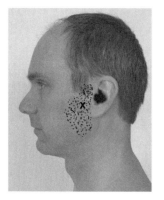

- Referred pain to your eyebrow, ear, jaw joint, mouth, and cheek region.

- Your upper or lower molars may be sensitive to pressure or temperature changes.

- You may have difficulty opening your mouth. (You should be able to fit the knuckles of the index and middle finger of your nondominant hand between your front teeth vertically.)

- Your jaw may deviate to one side when opening.

- You may have one-sided ringing or other noises in your ear, often described as a low roaring. If it occurs on both sides, fluctuation in its intensity is likely to be one-sided (as opposed to two-sided tinnitus, which is caused by factors other than trigger points, such as certain medications and noise damage).

- You may have pressure in your sinus area that feels like a sinus infection.

- You may have puffiness under your eye on the affected side due to restriction of blood flow from the area around your eyes.

- Your eyelid muscles may spasm.

- The masseter muscle may play a role in tension headaches.

Possible Causes and Perpetuators

Postural

- Head-forward posture

Medical or Structural

- Low thyroid function

- Anemia

- Vitamin deficiencies (especially B vitamins)

- Electrolyte imbalances (sodium, potassium, calcium, and magnesium)

- Chronic infections of any type, but particularly in or around your mouth

- Mouth breathing

- Trauma, such as prolonged overstretching during dental work

- Direct trauma from an accident

Other

- Depression, extreme emotional tension, or even moderate emotional tension (perhaps the most common cause)

- A high-stress job or relationship where you cannot safely express your feelings (for example, holding back anger or biting your tongue)

- Grinding your teeth (bruxism), which you may do only at night, when you aren't aware of it

- Changes in your bite, whether due to dental work, natural changes, or worn-out dentures

- Thumb sucking after infancy

- Chewing gum

- Clamping a pipe or cigarette holder in your teeth

- Constantly biting off threads when sewing

- Cracking nuts or ice between your teeth

- Activation of satellite trigger points by referral from trigger points in your sternocleido-mastoid or upper trapezius muscles

Helpful Hints

To learn proper posture and reduce head-forward posture, see "Head-Forward Posture" in chapter 5, Body Mechanics. Don't chew gum, or hold a pipe or cigarette holder clamped between your teeth. Avoid foods that require a lot of prolonged chewing or cracking of hard objects.

Since changes in your bite can be either the cause or the result of trigger points, it's best to first identify and relieve your trigger points before making permanent dental corrections. A splint or bite guard can help change your bite, or at least prevent you from grinding your teeth. Your dentist may have other solutions for your particular situation. Be sure to choose a dentist who has experience with trigger points and temporomandibular joint dysfunction, and who will take the time to make sure corrective devices fit properly. If these devices don't fit well, they can make trigger points worse and cause additional joint problems. If you must have a long dental procedure, see if your dentist is willing to give your mouth periodic rest breaks or use a bite block. Do the relevant self-treatments and stretches both before and after your appointment.

Difficulty opening your mouth may be due to trigger points in other muscles. If you can't find trigger points in your masseter or other mouth muscles, or if you've relieved them but still can't open your mouth fully, search for trigger points in your sternocleidomastoid and trapezius muscles.

Treat the cause of mouth breathing. Mechanical problems such as nasal polyps or a deviated septum may require surgery. Chronic sinusitis or allergies can be treated with acupuncture, herbs, or homeopathic remedies. Flushing your nasal passages with a warm saline solution may be helpful. You can use a Neti Pot, available at health food stores, to do this. Depending on the cause of the problem, a naturopathic doctor can use a small inflatable balloon to open up your nasal passages. For more information, see "Chronic Infections" in chapter 7, Other Perpetuating Factors.

Chronic infections of all kinds must be eliminated or controlled as best as possible, and the same is true of other medical and nutritional perpetuating factors. See a doctor or naturopath to determine if you have a low-functioning thyroid, anemia, a vitamin deficiency, or an electrolyte imbalance. A deficiency in calcium, magnesium, potassium, or sodium is easily remedied with supplements, which will usually relieve symptoms within one to two weeks.

If emotional factors are causing you to grind your teeth, see a counselor, learn relaxation and coping techniques, and otherwise work to reduce stress wherever possible.

Self-Help Techniques

Applying Pressure

Masseter Pressure

Using the hand opposite the side you're working on, insert your thumb inside your mouth but outside your gums. You may relax your jaw once your thumb is in place. With your index and middle fingers, press on the outside of your cheek, pinching your masseter between your fingers and thumb. Be sure to work all the way from the bottom of your jaw up to your cheekbone and all the way back toward your ear. See the anatomical drawing of the muscle at the start of the chapter so you'll know what you're aiming for.

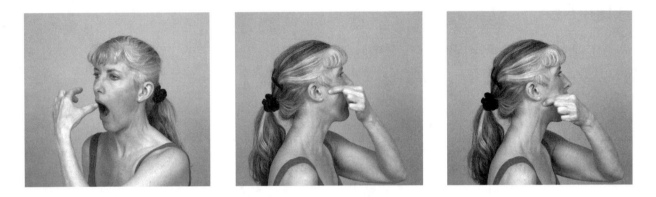

Stretches

Mouth Stretch

Warm your face with hot, moist towels if possible. Place one hand on your forehead and use two fingers of your other hand to gently pull your jaw forward and down. Count to eight and then relax. Repeat five to six times.

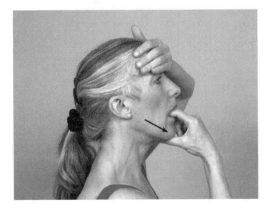
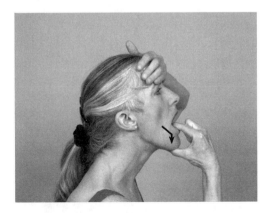

Exercises

Tongue Rolls

Tongue rolls help relax the muscles of the mouth. For complete instructions for this exercise, see the section "Abuse of Muscles" in chapter 5, Body Mechanics.

Yawning

Yawning is a good exercise to stretch and condition the masseter muscle.

Also See

- Chapter 13, Temporalis (satellite trigger points)
- Chapter 17, Medial Pterygoid (satellite trigger points)
- Chapter 12, Sternocleidomastoid
- Chapter 14, Facial and Scalp Muscles (satellite trigger points)
- Chapter 10, Trapezius

Conclusion

If you suspect masseter trigger points but were unable to relieve your symptoms with the self-help techniques in this chapter, you may need to see a dentist to rule out problems with your teeth or jaw joint disks. If you can't open your jaw due to spasms, you may need to see a doctor to rule out several types of infection or a tumor.

Chapter 16

Lateral Pterygoid

Trigger points in the lateral pterygoid are frequently the cause of the jaw not tracking properly, resulting in temporomandibular joint dysfunction. Dentists usually focus on treating this problem by working on the joint or teeth. However, if the problem is caused by trigger points in the muscles, this is ineffective.

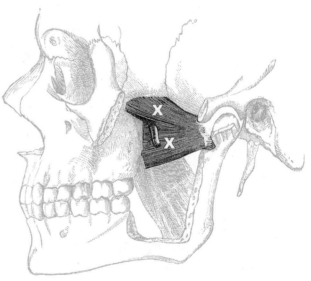

Common Symptoms

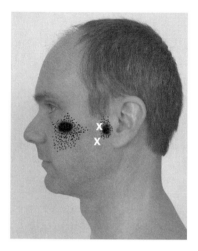

- Referred pain occurs deep in the temporomandibular joint and over your cheek.

- You may have pain with chewing.

- You may have a small amount of loss of range of motion, probably unnoticed.

- Your jaw may wobble back and forth when you open and close your mouth, usually deviating away from the side with trigger points.

- You may have tinnitus (ringing in the ears) in either one ear or both.

- Your nose may run, and because you might describe the referred pain as sinus pain, you could be misdiagnosed with sinusitis.

- Trigger points can be either the cause or the result of premature tooth contact, when one pair of teeth touches before the others do.

- If the buccal nerve becomes entrapped, you may have a weird tingling or numbness in your cheek.

Possible Causes and Perpetuators

Postural

- Head-forward posture

Medical or Structural

- Degenerative arthritis in the temporomandibular joint (which is not only a cause of trigger points, but can itself be caused by trigger points in the lateral pterygoid)

- Having one leg shorter than the other

- Having sit bones that aren't level because one side is smaller

- Deficiency of B vitamins, particularly folate

Activities

- Playing a wind instrument or the violin

Other

- Emotional tension, anxiety, or stress

- Trigger points in the sternocleidomastoid muscle

- Grinding your teeth

- Chewing gum or biting your nails excessively

- Premature tooth contact

- Thumb sucking after infancy

Helpful Hints

Look in a mirror, place the tip of your tongue as far back on the roof of your mouth as you can, and open your mouth. If you have the symptoms noted above and your jaw opens straight, the lateral pterygoid is the main culprit. If your jaw zigzags, other muscles in or around the mouth may also be involved, or you could have a problem with the temporomandibular joint itself and the lateral pterygoid may or may not be involved. You may need to get fitted for an occlusal splint. See your dentist. If there is no degeneration of the jaw joint itself, acupuncture is very successful with TMJ problems. Even if you do have degeneration or arthritis, acupuncture will still be helpful for pain control, but it won't restore the joint to its original condition.

To learn proper posture, see "Head-Forward Posture" in chapter 5, Body Mechanics. Get evaluated for any asymmetry in leg length or hemipelvis size, and get corrective lifts if necessary. Take a good B complex supplement, along with folic acid. Don't chew gum or eat foods that are too chewy or hard. Check for trigger points in your sternocleidomastoid, as they can cause satellite trigger points in the lateral pterygoid. If emotional factors are causing you to grind your teeth, see a counselor, learn relaxation and coping techniques, and otherwise work to reduce stress wherever possible.

Self-Help Techniques

Applying Pressure

Lateral Pterygoid Pressure

Using your index finger, place your finger between your cheek and your upper molars. Slide it all the way to the back, behind the last molar, and press in toward your nose. You will not be able to access the entire muscle, so it may be impossible for you to entirely eliminate its trigger points with self-treatment. Doing so may require the assistance of someone trained in trigger point injections specifically in this area, or acupuncture.

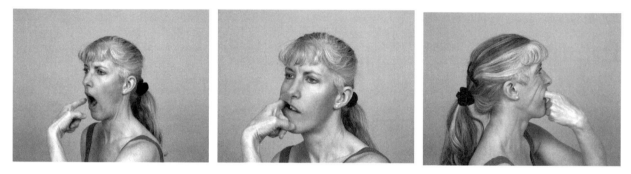

Stretches

Lateral Pterygoid Stretch

After applying a hot pack to your cheeks, lie down and rest your head against a firm support. Relax your jaw, gently push back on your chin with your fingers and gently and slowly rock your jawbone from side to side.

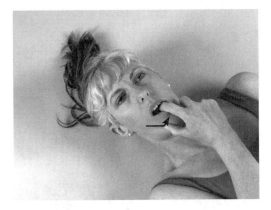 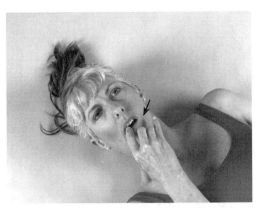

Next, increase your range of motion by jutting your jawbone out (away from your face) for a few seconds, and then pulling it back as far as you can, with no assistance from your fingers.

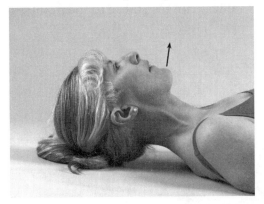 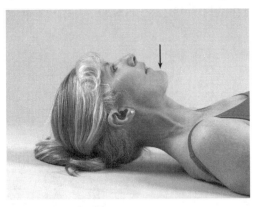

Finally, place your index finger on the inside of your lower teeth and your thumb under your jaw and gently pull down and forward.

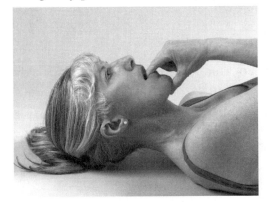 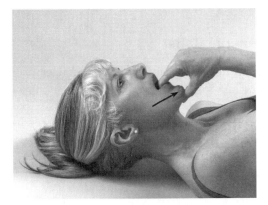

Exercises

Lateral Pterygoid Exercise

Once your lateral pterygoid trigger points have been inactivated for a few weeks, add resistance to the lateral pterygoid stretch above. When moving your jaw from side to side, gentle press your jaw against your fingers at the same time you are using your fingers to move the jaw to the opposite side.

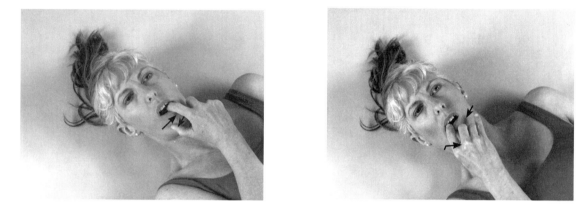

When jutting your jaw out, use one hand to gently apply some resistance to the point of your chin.

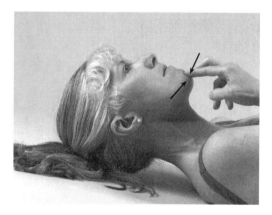

Tongue Rolls

Tongue rolls help relax the muscles of the mouth. For complete instructions for this exercise, see the section "Abuse of Muscles" in chapter 5, Body Mechanics.

Also See

- Chapter 17, Medial Pterygoid

- Chapter 15, Masseter

- Chapter 12, Sternocleidomastoid

Conclusion

The referred pain from lateral pterygoid trigger points can be confused with pain from the temporomandibular joint, but it doesn't have the more intense localized tenderness of joint inflammation. It also does not have the spasming electrical-type pain of tic douloureux. The referred pain tends to be more achy, and can be relieved with trigger point treatment, which the other causes cannot. Be sure to work on this muscle for at least a few weeks prior to getting any kind of dental intervention.

Chapter 17

Medial Pterygoid

Trigger points in the medial pterygoid alone are unlikely to cause headaches. However, when they occur in conjunction with trigger points in other chewing muscles and the muscles in the neck, they can contribute to TMJ problems and, indirectly, to headaches. The muscle is located behind the jawbone, which has been cut out in the anatomical drawing to allow a clear view.

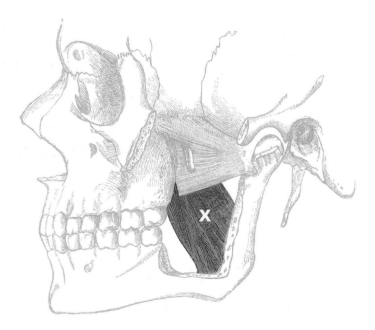

Common Symptoms

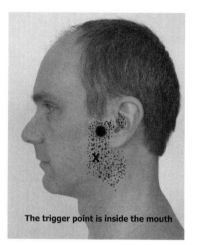

The trigger point is inside the mouth

- Pain is referred to the back of the mouth, tongue, and throat; below and around the jaw joint; and deep in the ear.

- You may have difficulty or pain with swallowing.

- You may feel like you have a sore throat.

- You may experience pain and some restriction when opening your jaw.

- You may experience pain when chewing or clenching your jaw.

- You may feel stuffiness in your ear if medial pterygoid trigger points prevent another muscle from opening the eustachian tubes.

- Usually you will only be able to open your mouth barely wide enough to insert the knuckles of the index and middle finger of your nondominant hand between your front teeth vertically; normally your mouth should open wide enough for almost three knuckles.

- If only one side has trigger points, your jaw may deviate to the same or opposite side when you open your mouth. This deviation mainly happens at the end of the movement.

Possible Causes and Perpetuators

Postural

- Head-forward posture

Other

- Trigger points in the lateral pterygoid

- Grinding or clenching your teeth

- Thumb sucking after infancy

- Chewing gum

- Improper bite alignment (which is not only a cause of trigger points, but can itself be caused by trigger points in the medial pterygoid)

- Anxiety, depression, and emotional tension

Helpful Hints

First, try eliminating trigger points in all your mouth and neck muscles. If you're having difficulty swallowing, try checking your sternocleidomastoid and digastric muscles for trigger points. If you clench your teeth, get fitted for a bite guard by a dentist. If your bite is off in a way that causes your teeth to make contact prematurely, try an occlusal splint. But before you're fitted for a dental appliance, try to inactivate any trigger points in the muscles in and around your mouth. Once they're inactivated, your bite may change. Also, consider chiropractic or osteopathic treatments, as your jaw may need an adjustment.

Get a pillow that won't place pressure on your jaw. These can usually be obtained at chiropractic offices.

Treat any chronic nutritional deficiencies (see chapter 6, Diet), as these can cause you to clench or grind your teeth. Identify and eliminate sources of anxiety, tension, and depression. Consider counseling, relaxation and coping techniques, and other self-help approaches. Acupuncture may be helpful, as it very successfully treats both TMJ problems and emotional tension.

If the above suggestions and trigger point treatments don't work, you may need to have a dentist adjust your bite, but this should be a last resort since it is irreversible.

Self-Help Techniques

Applying Pressure

Medial Pterygoid Pressure

Using the index finger of the hand opposite the side with the medial pterygoid trigger points, reach inside your mouth, inside your teeth, and all the way inside behind the upper molars, just behind the jaw joint. Sweep downward along the soft tissue behind your molars to the floor of your mouth. Press and hold anything that is tender. If this causes a gag reflex, take a deep breath and hold it while you're treating the trigger points.

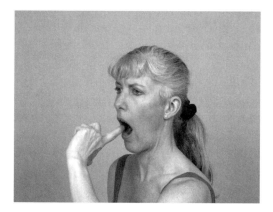 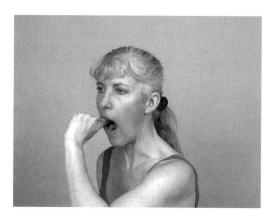

Stretches and Exercises

The stretches and exercises for the medial pterygoid are the same as those for the lateral pterygoid, in chapter 16.

Also See

- Chapter 18, Digastric

- Chapter 12, Sternocleidomastoid

- Chapter 16, Lateral Pterygoid

- Chapter 15, Masseter

Conclusion

Trigger points in the pectoralis major and pectoralis minor muscles may keep trigger points in the medial pterygoid active, so it is worthwhile to consider that there may be trigger points in these muscles that need to be relieved. Since they don't directly cause headaches or TMJ pain, the trigger points mentioned above are not addressed in this book, but if you can't relieve your symptoms with the self-help techniques in this book after six to eight weeks, you may wish to consider treating trigger points in the pectoral muscles. See the Resources section for books and other resources that can provide guidance on self-treatment of muscles not covered in this book.

Chapter 18

Digastric

As with the medial pterygoid, trigger points in the digastric muscle alone are unlikely to cause headaches. However, when they occur in conjunction with trigger points in other muscles in or around the mouth and the muscles in the neck, they can contribute to TMJ problems and, indirectly, to headaches.

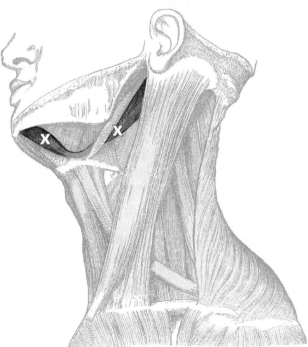

Common Symptoms

- The part of the muscle closest to the ear refers pain and tenderness below the ear and sometimes into the back of the skull, while the part beneath the chin refers pain to the four front lower teeth and just below those teeth.

- You may have difficulty swallowing or a sensation of a lump in your throat.

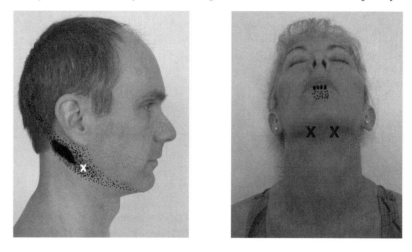

Possible Causes and Perpetuators

Medical or Structural

- Mouth breathing due to obstructions or other problems in your nasal passages can cause digastric trigger points.

- In the space below your earlobe is a little point of bone that can become calcified and lengthened (Eagle syndrome). Eagle syndrome can cause problems such as pain, dizziness, and blurred vision on the affected side, especially when your head is turned all the way to the affected side. The bone can cause and perpetuate trigger points in the posterior belly of the digastric and the medial pterygoid. The dizziness and blurred vision may be caused by trigger points formed in the sternocleidomastoid. Pressure against the carotid artery when turning your head may cause part of the pain, as well as dizziness.

Other

- Grinding your teeth or jutting your jaw out

- Trigger points in your masseter or sternocleidomastoid muscles

Helpful Hints

Because referral from the posterior portion of the digastric is easy to confuse with referral from the sternocleidomastoid muscle, check your sternocleidomastoid first. If treating trigger points in your sternocleidomastoid isn't effective, then check the digastric for trigger points and work on them. Work on your masseter and temporalis muscles, particularly on the *opposite* side.

Don't chew gum or eat foods that are too chewy or hard. If emotional factors are causing you to grind your teeth, see a counselor, learn relaxation and coping techniques, and otherwise work to reduce stress wherever possible.

Treat the cause of mouth breathing. Mechanical problems such as nasal polyps or a deviated septum may require surgery. Chronic sinusitis or allergies can be treated with acupuncture, herbs, or homeopathic remedies. Flushing your nasal passages with a warm saline solution may be helpful. You can use a Neti Pot, available at health food stores, to do this. Naturopathic doctors can use a small inflatable balloon to open up your nasal passages. For more information, see "Chronic Infections" in chapter 7, Other Perpetuating Factors.

If the above suggestions don't work, you may need to have a dentist adjust your bite, but this should be a last resort since it is irreversible. If you have the symptoms of Eagle syndrome, described above, you will need to have the area X-rayed for confirmation and possibly have the bone surgically removed.

Self-Help Techniques

Applying Pressure

Digastric Pressure

Hook your thumb under the rim of your jaw and push toward the top of your head (pic. 1). Start in the front and work your way back, working around the back angle of your jaw below your earlobe.

Once you get around the back angle of your jawbone (pic. 2), press your thumb toward your nose (pic. 3). It will be easier to treat this portion of the muscle if you deviate your jaw toward the side on which you're working. *Do not push deeply into your neck muscles*, particularly in the area below your earlobe, as you can break the bony little point.

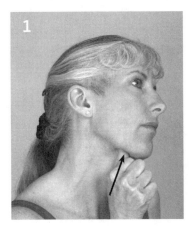 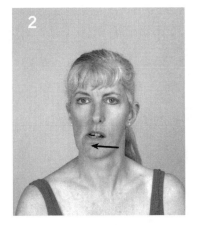 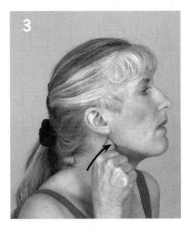

Stretches

Mouth Stretch

See chapter 15, Masseter, for details on how to do this stretch.

Exercises

Digastric Exercise

Once your trigger points have been inactivated for a few weeks, you can do the following exercise. Lie face-up with your mouth open less than halfway. While slowly moving your jawbone from side to side, use your hand to apply gentle resistance on the side you're moving toward.

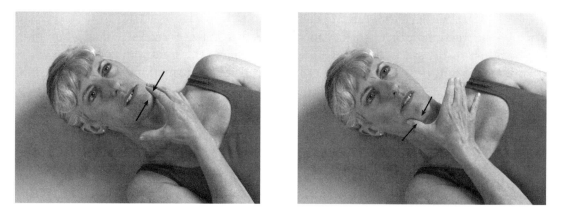

Tongue Rolls

Tongue rolls help relax the muscles of the mouth. For complete instructions for this exercise, see the section "Abuse of Muscles" in chapter 5, Body Mechanics.

Also See

- Chapter 12, Sternocleidomastoid

- Chapter 13, Temporalis

- Chapter 15, Masseter

Conclusion

Difficulty swallowing, pain when you talk, a mysterious sore throat, and pain in your head, neck, throat, tongue, or mouth may be caused by other muscles deep in the front of your neck. You would need to see a practitioner trained in deep anterior neck muscles in order to explore the possibility of trigger points in these muscles.

Appendix A

A Word About Fibromyalgia

When pain is widespread, it is usually given the diagnosis of fibromyalgia or myofascial pain syndrome. When I see bodywide pain and tender points, I wonder what is going on systemically; that is, what could be affecting the body as a whole? Anemia, hormonal imbalances (including menopause), nutritional deficiencies, hypoglycemia, and allergies are examples of conditions that could cause or contribute to this sort of widespread tenderness.

What Is Fibromyalgia?

Allopathic (Western) medicine defines fibromyalgia as a chronic disorder associated with widespread muscle and soft-tissue pain, tenderness, and fatigue. Diagnosis is made by pressing eighteen areas to check for tenderness, and if at least eleven of the points are tender and the pain has been present for at least three months, the person is diagnosed positive for fibromyalgia. Treatment usually involves some kind of pain medication and counseling for chronic pain management.

Most of the recent Western research has indicated that the cause may possibly be some sort of bodywide metabolic and neurochemical problem, including deficiency of the neurotransmitter serotonin (Simons, Travell, and Simons 1999). This deficiency causes an increase in pain sensitivity and a higher concentration of substance P (a compound involved in the regulation of the pain threshold) in the spinal fluid.

Although allopathic medicine has not found a definitive cause for fibromyalgia, someone with the same symptoms whose skin also feels spongy to the touch would, in terms of a traditional Chinese medicine diagnosis, be diagnosed with damp-heat or damp-cold in the muscles. Although there isn't a one-to-one correlation between allopathic and traditional Chinese medicine diagnoses for any disease, in cases of what I consider true fibromyalgia (in the allopathic sense), the tissues will feel somewhat spongy to the touch. Dampness easily combines with heat or cold, and typically fibromyalgia is aggravated by either hot or cold weather, or the application of heat or cold. People with fibromyalgia typically feel better in a drier climate, since a damp climate can aggravate the condition.

A damp-producing diet can cause or perpetuate fibromyalgia; for lists of foods to avoid and foods that will be beneficial, see "Foods and Drinks to Avoid Based on Pain Type" in chapter 6, Diet. The digestive system is responsible for transforming fluids, and if it isn't working well, you will tend to accumulate dampness in various body parts. For some people, that is in the muscle layer of the body. Acupuncture and damp-draining herbs and foods are very successful in treating fibromyalgia, as long as the practitioner is careful not to overtreat the patient. Massage with light to moderate pressure will likely help with the acute pain, but it won't resolve the underlying conditions causing fibromyalgia.

If you have fibromyalgia, the book *Fibromyalgia and Chronic Myofascial Pain: A Survival Manual*, by Devin Starlanyl and Mary Ellen Copeland (2001), is an excellent resource. It provides an in-depth look at the physiology of the condition from a Western perspective and discusses the concept of interstitial edema, which I believe correlates to the traditional Chinese medicine concept of damp-heat or damp-cold in the muscles. Interstitial edema is a condition in which excess interstitial fluid builds up in the body's "interstitial space," or "third space." It's neither inside the cells nor outside the cells, so the structure of the interstitial space is hard to visualize, but within this "in between" space, various substances are transferred between blood and lymph *through* the interstitial space. Lymph fluid, which is composed of interstitial fluid, brings cells substances that they need and carries away excess liquid and metabolic waste. If something interferes with the flow of lymph, such as lack of exercise, improper breathing, constipation, or muscle tightness and restricted range of motion, excessive amounts of fluid and metabolic waste can become trapped in the interstitial space, leading to swelling of the tissues (Starlanyl and Copeland 2001). The authors believe that it is these swollen tissues that cause the pain and tenderness associated with fibromyalgia.

Fibromyalgia Symptoms Versus Trigger Points

In addition to tender points, most fibromyalgia patients also have at least some trigger points (and probably numerous trigger points), but there are distinct differences between the tender points of fibromyalgia and trigger points. Trigger points restrict range of motion, whereas too great a range of motion is common with fibromyalgia. With trigger points, usually only the trigger point itself is tender, whereas people with fibromyalgia experience pain pretty much everywhere to some degree. In addition to having tender points, about 75 percent of people with fibromyalgia also feel fatigued, don't feel rested upon waking, and are stiff in the morning (Simons, Travell, and Simons 1999).

In spite of the differences in symptoms, treating trigger points can help treat the pain of fibromyalgia. You probably won't be able to tell the difference between a trigger point and a tender point when you're applying pressure, so use the referral pattern photos and the symptom lists in the muscle chapters (chapters 10 through 18) to help you figure out where a trigger point is likely to be located, and then treat that muscle.

Conclusion

If you have fibromyalgia and receive trigger point injections, pain relief will not be immediate due to postinjection soreness, which can last from nine to twenty days (for those without fibromyalgia, postinjection soreness only lasts a day or two). Treatment of trigger points by a professional, in combination with the self-help techniques in this book, will help manage the pain associated with fibromyalgia. However, you also need to address the underlying causes and perpetuating factors in order to obtain lasting relief. Long-term dietary changes will help immensely.

Appendix B

A Special Note to Therapists Teaching Self-Help Techniques

Be sure to explain trigger points and referral patterns to your patients. Tell them why you are working on an area that is different than where they've indicated they feel symptoms. If a patient is expecting a full-body massage but also seeks treatment for specific problems, explain that there won't be time to fit in an entire full-body massage in addition to specific treatments. If a patient has pain in many areas, recommend that they choose a few areas to work on in each visit.

At the beginning of every visit, have your patients color in a body chart to show their symptoms and intensity (see chapter 9 for a blank body chart). Some will be resistant to doing this, saying "It's just the same." Since many patients improve slowly, their perception may be that their symptoms are the same when in fact the area affected is smaller or the pain is less intense or less frequent. And if indeed their symptoms haven't changed, then you know that you are missing the trigger points, that the patient is missing the trigger points when doing self-treatments, or that perpetuating factors need to be addressed. Also, sometimes patients will announce that they have a new problem when in fact it's an old problem that they've just forgotten about. It is important to have a historical record.

While you are working on a patient, ask them about their pain with questions such as these: "Does this feel familiar, like the way it feels when you press on it with the ball?" "Is this less tender than last time?" "Are you feeling better, the same, or worse?" Sometimes when they fill out body charts, they'll mark the same area with the same intensity and frequency of pain but actually report feeling much better, so you can't go strictly by the numbers. You may need to educate patients about why you need to ask questions during treatment: so that you can get feedback on invoked referral patterns and pressure-pain levels, and also gather information about potential perpetuating factors and other information critical to providing the best treatment possible.

I keep a master checklist of muscles for each patient so I can easily refer to it while working on that patient, circling the involved muscles and writing short comments. I look at the trigger point referral charts and ask myself which muscles might harbor trigger points that are causing the person's pain.

If you have read about or been trained in trigger point therapy, you've probably heard about eliciting the twitch response and jump sign as a diagnostic criterion. While this may be important for a doctor who is sticking a hypodermic needle into a patient and must do so accurately and in a limited number of places, as a massage therapist or physical therapist you are not under the same constraints. It is even questionable whether the absence of these signs or the inability of the practitioner to invoke them rules out the diagnosis of a trigger point. Since eliciting a twitch response and a jump sign can cause a great deal of pain, this can cause the patient to tense up and stay tense in anticipation of further unexpected pain-inducing moves on your part. Skilled therapists can locate trigger points without these diagnostic criteria, in part because they are massaging over an area larger than the tip of a needle, and also because they have the option of working on several trigger points in a session. When you learn to palpate trigger points and gather the right information from the patient, you can locate trigger points without causing more discomfort than the patient can easily tolerate.

Ask patients if they'd like to learn self-help techniques, and if they would, explain that you'll need to save five to ten minutes at the end of the treatment to do so (and longer the first time). Explain that people who do self-treatments get better much faster. At the beginning of the first self-help session, briefly go over the basic self-help guidelines verbally, give them printed instructions that cover those basics, and ask patients to read through the guidelines again before they do self-treatments the first time. Tell them to start the next day, so the techniques and guidelines will still be fresh in their mind. Give them pictures of the muscles they'll be treating, and use a highlighting marker to emphasize the most important things for them to remember.

Demonstrate the self-treatment you want the patient to do, and then watch them do it. This will help the patient understand the technique much better. It will also make them more likely to do the self-treatments, since even a few moments of practicing will help them realize that self-treatment really will help; as a result, they'll look forward to doing it. Only teach two new self-help techniques per visit, prioritizing your selection depending on what the patient needs to work on; any more than two is probably too much for patients to remember. Patients are far more likely to start doing the self-help if they can leave your office with the necessary equipment. Keep a supply of tennis balls, golf balls, racquetballs, and baseballs in your office for patients to purchase.

On subsequent visits, find out if the patient is doing the self-treatments, where they are doing it, how often, how much pressure they used and whether it felt too hard or too soft, whether there were any problems, and so on. You may need to review the techniques with them again. It's a lot of information, and the concepts will be new to most people. If a patient is having problems locating the areas on which they need to work, mark it on them with a permanent marker (which lasts three to four days), or give them a landmark. Palpate the muscle tissues to see if they are improving. If the tissues haven't softened, then it is likely they are missing the correct areas, even if they think they are locating them accurately. Walk them through it again, or figure out a different way they can access the area if what they've been doing isn't working. If they aren't doing the self-treatments, find out why. Often people stop doing the self-treatments because it was too painful. Reiterate that they need to figure out how to make the self-help less painful, such as starting on a bed, a pillow, or a folded-up blanket when using pressure against a ball. If they simply don't want to do self-treatments, consider that you may just want to work on them and not teach them something they aren't going to do. If patients ask what they can do to help their symptoms improve more quickly, reiterate that addressing any perpetuating factors and doing self-treatments are the best things they can do to resolve the problem.

Conclusion

Above all, be patient with your patients! For most of them, learning about trigger points involves a lot of new information, especially if they aren't familiar with anatomy. Patients may need to be walked through the self-help techniques and be reminded more than once to do them. Some people will expect you to "fix" them and won't do anything to help themselves. For those people, I do the best I can and let go of the goal of them getting better as fast as I think they could. And when working with patients who *are* willing to help themselves, the rewards are tremendous.

Resources

Balch, J. F., and P. A. Balch. 2000. *Prescription for Nutritional Healing: A Practical A-Z Reference to Drug-Free Remedies Using Vitamins, Minerals, Herbs and Food Supplements.* New York: Avery.

DeLaune, Valerie, LAC. 2004. *Pain Relief with Trigger Point Self-Help* (compact disc). Juneau, AK: Available at www.triggerpointrelief.com.

DeLaune, Valerie, LAC. 2008. Trigger Point Therapy for Headaches, Migraines, and TMJ Pains. Videos of Self-Treatment Techniques (compact disc). Jeneau, AK. Available at www.triggerpoint relief.com

Davies, Clair. 2004. *The Trigger Point Therapy Workbook.* 2nd edition. Oakland, CA: New Harbinger Publications.

Simons, D. G., J. G. Travell, and L. S. Simons. 1999. *Myofascial Pain and Dysfunction: The Trigger Point Manual.* Vol. 1, *The Upper Extremities.* 2nd ed. Baltimore: Lippincott Williams & Wilkins.

Starlanyl, D., and M. E. Copeland. 2001. *Fibromyalgia and Chronic Myofascial Pain: A Survival Manual.* 2nd ed. Oakland, CA: New Harbinger Publications.

Travell, J. G., and D. G. Simons. 1992. *Myofascial Pain and Dysfunction: The Trigger Point Manual.* Vol. 2, *The Lower Extremities.* Baltimore: Lippincott Williams & Wilkins.

Websites

Triggerpointrelief.com. Author's website with additional resources, articles, and links to helpful sites.

The Pressure Positive Company. This company sells self-pressure devices and massage tools. Their website has an information center with articles and links to other helpful sites. 800-603-5107. www.pressurepositive.com.

New Harbinger Publications. New Harbinger publishes books on a variety of self-help topics which you may find helpful. 800-748-6273. www.newharbinger.com.

Superfeet. This company sells noncorrective footbeds, and their website can help you locate a dealer who can make Superfeet custom footbeds for you. 800-634-6618. www.superfeet.com.

Acupuncture Today. This online publication is searchable by topic, and you may be able to determine whether your medical condition is treatable with acupuncture. www.acupuncturetoday.com.

Massage Today. This online publication is searchable by topic, and you may be able to determine whether your medical condition is treatable with massage. www.massagetoday.com.

References

American Medical Association. 1989. *The American Medical Association Encyclopedia of Medicine: An A-to-Z Reference Guide to Over 5,000 Medical Terms Including Symptoms, Diseases, Drugs and Treatments.* New York: Random House.

Audette, J. F., F. Wang, and H. Smith. 2004. Bilateral activation of motor unit potentials with unilateral needle stimulation of active myofascial trigger points. *American Journal of Physical Medicine and Rehabilitation* 83(5):368-74.

Balch, J. F., and P. A. Balch. 2000. *Prescription for Nutritional Healing: A Practical A-Z Reference to Drug-Free Remedies Using Vitamins, Minerals, Herbs and Food Supplements.* New York: Avery.

Bendtsen, L. 2000. Central sensitization in tension-type headache—possible pathophysiological mechanisms. *Cephalalgia: An International Journal of Headache* 20(5):486-508.

Borg-Stein, J., and D. G. Simons. 2002. Myofascial pain. *Archives of Physical Medicine and Rehabilitation* 83(Suppl 1):S40-47.

Calandre, E. P., J. Hidalgo, J. M. Garcia-Leiva, and F. Rico-Villadermoros. 2006. Trigger point evaluation in migraine patients: An indication of peripheral sensitization linked to migraine predisposition? *European Journal of Neurology* 13(3):244-49.

Cleveland Clinic. 2007. Overview of headaches in adults. www.clevelandclinic.org/health/healthinfo/docs/2500/2556.asp?index=9639.

Edwards, J., and N. Knowles. 2003. Superficial dry needling and active stretching in the treatment of myofascial pain—a randomised controlled trial. *Acupuncture in Medicine* 21(3):80-86.

Graff-Radford, S. B., and A. Newman. 2004. Obstructive sleep apnea and cluster headaches. *Headache: The Journal of Head and Face Pain* 44(6):607-10.

Healthcommunities.com. 2002. Headache: Overview, types, incidence and prevalence, causes. www.neurologychannel.com/headache.

Jensen, R., and J. Olesen. 1996. Initiating mechanisms of experimentally induced tension-type headache. *Cephalalgia: An International Journal of Headache* 16(3):175-82.

Kemper, J. T., Jr., and J. P. Okeson. 1983. Craniomandibular disorders and headaches. *Journal of Prosthetic Dentistry* 49(5):702-5.

Marcus, D. A., L. Scharff, S. Mercer, and D. C. Turk. 1999. Musculoskeletal abnormalities in chronic headache: A controlled comparison of headache diagnostic groups. *Headache: The Journal of Head and Face Pain* 39(1):21-27.

Olesen, J. 1991. Clinical and pathophysiological observations in migraine and tension-type headache explained by integration of vascular, supraspinal and myofascial inputs. *Pain* 46(2):125-32.

Packard, R. C. 2002. The relationship of neck injury and post-traumatic headache. *Current Pain and Headache Reports* 6(4):301-7.

Schoenen, J., J. Jacquy, and M. Lenaerts. 1998. Effectiveness of high-dose riboflavin in migraine prophylaxis: A randomized controlled trial. *Neurology* 50(2):466-70.

Simons, D. G. 2003. Enigmatic trigger points often cause enigmatic musculoskeletal pain. Presentation at the STAR Symposium, Columbus, Ohio, May 22. Available at http://ergonomics.osu.edu/pdfs/2003%20STAR%20Symposium/Simons%20Trigger.pdf.

———. 2004. Review of enigmatic MTrPs as a common cause of enigmatic musculoskeletal pain and dysfunction. *Journal of Electromyography and Kinesiology* 14(1):95-107.

Simons, D. G., J. G. Travell, and L. S. Simons. 1999. *Myofascial Pain and Dysfunction: The Trigger Point Manual.* Vol. 1, *The Upper Extremities.* 2nd ed. Baltimore: Lippincott Williams & Wilkins.

Starlanyl, D., and M. E. Copeland. 2001. *Fibromyalgia and Chronic Myofascial Pain: A Survival Manual.* 2nd ed. Oakland, CA: New Harbinger Publications.

Travell, J. G., and D. G. Simons. 1983. *Myofascial Pain and Dysfunction: The Trigger Point Manual.* Baltimore: Lippincott Williams & Wilkins.

———. 1992. *Myofascial Pain and Dysfunction: The Trigger Point Manual.* Vol. 2, *The Lower Extremities.* Baltimore: Lippincott Williams & Wilkins.

Treaster, D., W. S. Marras, D. Burr, J. E. Sheedy, and D. Hart. 2006. Myofascial trigger point development from visual and postural stressors during computer work. *Journal of Electromyography and Kinesiology* 16(2):115-24.

Index

Valerie DeLaune, L.Ac., is a licensed acupuncturist and certified neuromuscular therapist, with a master's degree in acupuncture from the Northwest Institute of Acupuncture and Oriental Medicine and a bachelor of science degree from the University of Washington. She holds professional certificates from the Heartwood Institute and the Brenneke School of Massage. She authors books and articles on trigger points and acupuncture topics and currently practices acupuncture in Juneau, AK. www.triggerpointrelief.com

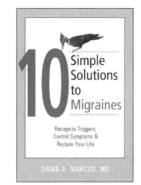
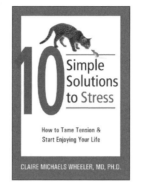
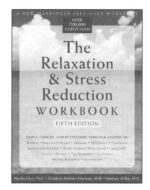
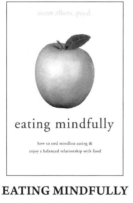
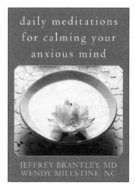
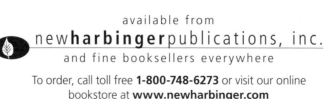